An Apple a Day........

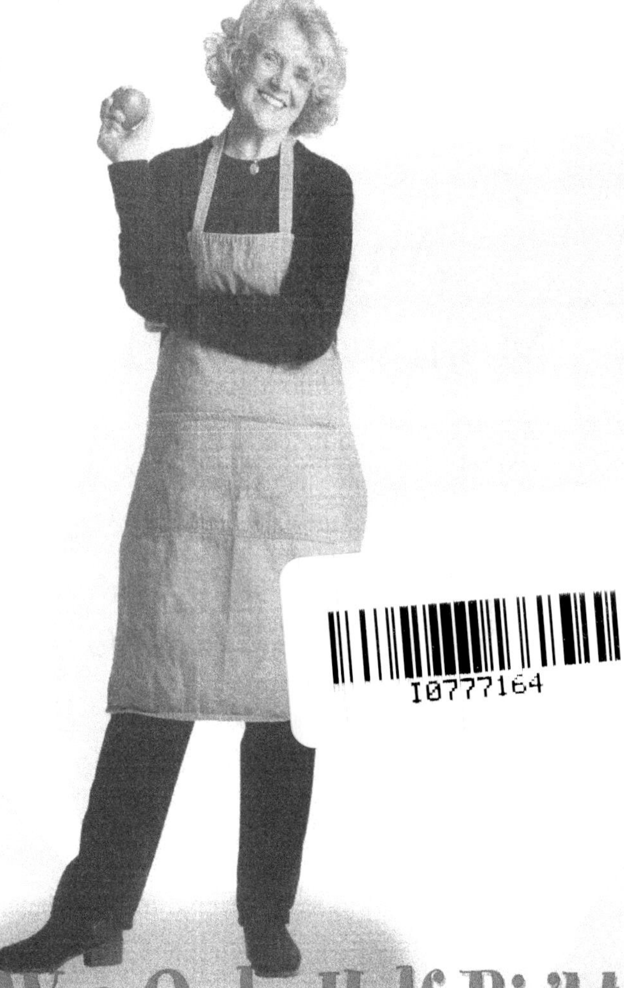

Mom Was Only Half Right

The Complete Health Story

by Emmanuel X. Enderlein

An Apple a Day –
Mom was Only Half Right

*The Complete Story
of Health, Water,
Fiber, Weight loss,
Constipation, and
Chronic Diarrhea.*

by

Emmanuel X. Enderlein

Dedication

To my friend, Alex, who fought colon cancer for ten years. When presented with this information, his response was, first a look of concern, sorrow and then relief, "Why didn't anyone tell me this?" He then requested that I write this book.

Alexander A. Araco

May 4, 1930 – September 16, 2001

Manufactured in the United
States of America

ISBN 13: 9781979920384

Preface

I long thought there was a missing link to health. Like everyone else, I was confused when I listened and read the information from the media. One day something is a cure; the next day it causes cancer. This scenario has been going on for my entire life.

I was raised in a military academy from the age of twelve, and went on to college and graduated. After college, I enlisted in the Air Force, and as an enlistee, K. P. (kitchen patrol) was inevitable. This experience proved to be one of the most enlightening of my life.

Among my assigned kitchen duties was dispensing salads and desserts at the end of the chow line. My enlightening observations were simply this. The personnel, male or female, whose plates consisted of vegetables usually small helpings of meat and potatoes always asked for a large salad and had fruit instead of cake for dessert. Those individuals were trim, appeared fit, and had great complexions.

On the other hand, the personnel whose plates consisted of extra meat and were piled high with mashed potatoes and no vegetables skipped the salad, but always went for the sweet cake. Most were heavier, un-shapely, with bad complexions.

I adjusted my own habits to eat healthier with good results.

Fast-forwarding twenty-five years, and I still was adhering to the same principles and still disliked broccoli, but fast foods had started to creep in and constipation was becoming a problem. I related this to age and just continued with laxatives. However, I was starting to become alarmed at all the medical problems that suddenly were engulfing our country. At this point I thought an exercise program might be the answer, so I started to run and lost 30 lbs., but I still lacked energy. In fact, some days my tired feeling never went away. I thought vitamins might help, so I took everything from mega doses of vitamin C to spirulina powder (a plant protein for more energy) – without results.

I then started to look at solving constipation with two natural products – a commercial fiber called psyllium seed husks and a natural laxative, prunes. It worked with some success, but I wondered why. What was the bottom line? How does all this work?

A dear friend, whose husband was operated on for colon cancer, suggested to me, that I research constipation at Jefferson Medical Library in Philadelphia. Later that week at a banquet, by a twist of fate, I found myself seated alongside a colo-rectal specialist, who suggested researching the studies of Dr. Trowell and Dr. Burkitt.

Shortly after, I read a newly released publication of a 937-page, 2002 federal government study on our diets. A reporter for the *Philadelphia Inquirer* summed up this information with the following comment **"It seems to me that it's telling us to consume more fiber."**

That was it – no explanations, nothing.

Reading a statement like that is almost like arriving at the edge of the cliff and no one, but no one, wants to jump into the unknown. There are a few exceptions, Paul Newman and Robert Redford did it in "Butch Cassidy and the Sundance Kid." Katie Couric did by televising her colonoscopy.

For us, the unknown is the colon – a six foot organ in our bodies, similar to a bicycle inner tube that defines our quality of life.

. . **really!**

This book explains why most never jump. From parents, to the media, from doctors to pharmaceutical companies. It's the only book containing detailed information written in layman terms, that thoroughly explains the problem and then solves it from the beginning to . . . End.

The rewards....Quality of Life and Life Itself

Acknowledgements

I would like to thank the people who had input into this book. My wife, Verne who just listened. My daughter's Kirsten and Dale and sister Gretchen, who became users of insoluble fiber and then believers. My good friend Gene Scarpa, who always lived the program.

CONTENTS

1- The Family and How We're Taught

Discovering why constipation is a problem

Whether you realize it or not, it starts in the family. Can you remember having a hard time eliminating in the morning before school? Perhaps you remember straining and pushing, knowing that you would feel a whole heck of a lot better if you did. Maybe you strained so hard that blood appeared, because those stomach pains were causing a lot of discomfort. In fact, it seemed that everything was stuck.

The embarrassing remedies

What do I do? If I ask Mom, it's guaranteed I'll get a laxative, which will cause classroom embarrassment at school. Or maybe it's the proven enema, which is worse because Mom gives it and I can't control it. Anyway, this was the scenario early on, with no advice on how to make my problem go away.

As I got older, and asked questions about constipation, I might get the stock parental answers. "Make sure you chew your food real well, vegetables are really good for you, especially broccoli. Drink plenty of juice and water or there is a laxative on the shelf in the bathroom." Think about it! The most important function of your life besides breathing and you get a sentence of advice or a laxative.

But why?

. . . Because constipation is never discussed, results are never shared and all terms pertaining to the condition are considered taboo. Try to engage family or friends in discussions on the topic. I guarantee it won't last a minute. Compare this to conversation on other topics such as, heart disease, cancer, weight loss, religion, music, politics, cars, or computers.....

If we communicated information on rockets the way we do on constipation, my guess is mankind would have never set off the first firecracker. Information on constipation has never advanced past the individual or the first generation in practical shared experience and knowledge.

2- The Medical Profession

Discovering the doctors' role in constipation

In 1971 words such as fiber, cellulose or roughage could not be found in any textbook of nutrition, medicine, surgery, gastroenterology or any medical journal (Preston, 1974, p.4) [End Notes 1]

Into the 1950s and beyond

According to research by Dr. Rudolph Ballentine, M.D., there were revolutionary writings on how a stagnant colon could affect health. However, our diets composed of fresh vegetables, fruits and unaltered feed for livestock were basically sound. The sense of urgency just didn't exist and interest disappeared. [End Notes 2]

In the 1960s and 1970s, our food supply started to change quickly, with food processing companies using preservatives, artificial flavoring, sweeteners and growth hormones for livestock. Dietary fiber (bran, the outside of wheat grain) was removed for ease of manufacturing, appearance, taste and profit. Fast food outlets and convenience stores were becoming the norm.

Health problems exploded

The medical profession changed to meet the multiple health issues. Gone was the family doctor, the generalist, who was replaced with a specialist. Mom now just purchased a laxative or medicine as advertised on TV.

The missing specialists

The question now becomes, if you are a very bright and gifted person, the top of your class, the valedictorian, would you really consider this area of the body for a prestigious career? I know my answer at that age. What's yours? Further validation is provided by Dr. Ballentine in his book, *Radical Healing*, quote "There seems to be a huge void in the literature where I should find mention of accumulation of waste in the body." [End Notes 3]

Only a few wanted to go there...

3- **Billions from Laxatives, Pain and Vitamins**

Discovering the monies at stake

The trip to corporate America

The next time you visit a drug store or chain store pharmacy; check out the aisle on laxatives. It's enormous – four shelves high, 15 to 20 feet long, and containing at least 15 brand names. It's selling the **fiber that was removed or we neglected to eat** for bulking/expanding the colon and a water substitute for flowability for water we didn't drink. This aisle is duplicated in every community nationwide and accounts for $2 billion in sales per year – guaranteed!

What else?

In the next aisle over, check out all the remedies for nagging headaches, upset stomachs or excessive gas, which are the effects of constipation (lack of fiber and moisture.) Or take a look at the aisle that contains vitamins to correct our low energy, which is really trying to correct the poisonous effect of constipation. Chalk up another $7 billion per year!

The real problem

Let me clarify. The stuff that we have eaten, steroids in poultry and beef, food additives and chemicals, have taken too long to exit our body and are still attached to the colon wall, stagnating, rotting, and causing 95% of our health problems. You might think that, with all the money we spend on drugs and medical advice, we deserve a number printed on the packaging so we can call to obtain a clear explanation of the problem.

Not with all the cash at stake

4- The Media

Handling all that information

Watching TV

Isn't it interesting how every newscaster brings us the health problem of the week? You know, the ones about obesity, and then a film clip of stomachs and rear ends, or the colonoscopy, pictures of the colon probe, or a female pressed up against the cold surface of an x-ray machine for a breast exam. Yet, in all their efforts to inform us, they never mention, or simply breeze through the fast food connection to health, at risk of offending the program sponsors.

The channels' doctors

If we have a celebrity, politician or VIP with a life threatening illness, then we have a local specialist telling us about the condition. Then the statistics of how many people die each year, recommending that if we have any symptoms we should see our doctor.

Missing the most important interview

How about the best health opportunity of all? We've all waited for the interview. You know the one, where the local newsie asks the 100 year birthday geezer or geezerette, "What's the secret to your health?" Well, the ego takes over, the 15 minutes of fame syndrome kicks in, and the centenarian answers, "I have a shot of whiskey and a cigar every day." When the honest and accurate answer should be "It's simple, I eat the right stuff, plenty of fiber, fruits and vegetables, . . .

To move my bowels one to two times per day

5- Constipation: What is it?

The dictionary's meaning of constipation: To crowd or pack together; difficulty or straining to evacuate.

Constipation/poor health really is.....

. . . insufficient water and fiber in the colon, causing food to spend more than 48 hours there. The feces lack the flowability and softness to negotiate the difficult 90-, 180-, 270-, and 360-degree turns, physical obstructions, and residue left in the colon from the past and distant past.

And chronic diarrhea is....

. . . A condition where intestinal parasites or bacterial infection, located in the residue left on the colon wall, grow and thrive due to a **fiberless history**. The colon is continually trying to rid itself of the irritation. It is behaving like a few laxatives, which work on the irritation principle.

Visualize the colon as an old deflated balloon, which folds back on itself because it lacks air to keep its shape. In the colon, lack of fiber and water for shape, lead to folds in which parasites and infections prosper.

48 hours and why it matters

Most cooked food, raw meats and unrefrigerated milk

spoils within 48 hours if left on your counter top at room temperature. [End Notes 4] The food that lingers more than 48 hours in your colon should be considered raw sewage. The toxins caused by this sewage now contaminate your body's **primary water supply, the colon.** The colon is the body's well, supplying 90% of all water needed. If it is full of toxins/chemicals, then water that filters through the sewage contaminates the bloodstream, creating 95% of non-infectious health problems.

48 hours stated another way

The math: a high-fiber, 12" to 18" long stool, eliminated 1 to 2 times a day is about 3 feet of feces per day. The colon is 6 feet long, so transit time is 48 hours.

Dr. Hugh Trowell indicated that, by passing a bulky, high-fiber stool, two to three times a day, the following common non- infective diseases disappeared. [End Notes 5]

- Crohn's disease
- Colorectal cancer
- Chronic diarrhea
- Coronary artery disease
- Breast cancer
- Varicose veins
- Diverticular disease
- Colon polyps
- Anemia
- Obesity
- Hypertension (high blood pressure)
- Irritable bowel syndrome

- Gallstones
- Rheumatoid arthritis
- Renal stones
- Hiatal hernia
- Gout
- Hypoparathyroidism
- Paget's disease
- Thyrotoxicosis
- Appendicitis

- Diabetes Type II
- Ulcerative colitis
- Dental problems
- Hashimoto's thyroiditis
- Multiple sclerosis
- Myasthenia gravis
- Pulmonary embolism
- Hemorrhoids
- Pernicious anemia (defective production of red blood cells, poor absorption of vitamin B)

Note: This list does not include conditions caused by new food additives. Definitions and symptoms of many of these conditions are provided in the Appendix of this book.

Findings are supported

From clinical necropsy data (examination of bodies after death) and 23 literature citations and personal communications involving five continents Dr. Trowell and Dr. Burkitt (1981) concluded that, with diets rich in fiber, people **rarely suffered** from the preceding list of health problems. [End Notes 6] Rich in fiber means 25 to 35 grams of insoluble fiber per day, every day!

This is a conclusion by experts, Dr. Trowell and Dr. Burkitt, the best in their field, the Dr. Salk's or Einstein's of fiber!

The information above is worth reading and rereading. Ask yourself questions such as: With our health crises, why isn't this information in newspapers, billboards, TV, and radio? Why isn't it discussed in grade schools, middle schools, and high schools? Why isn't it printed on prescription drug containers and included in hospital and insurance bills?

THE QUESTION ALWAYS ASKED

"This ailment (colon cancer, heart disease, etc.) has been in my family for years. In fact, even my aunt and uncle have it, so why does a high-fiber diet help?"

THE ANSWER

In a lot of cases, you may have only inherited your parents' eating habits – Mom's cooking, Dad's favorite restaurants, and fast foods. That's why you see the obese kids with the obese parents.

6- Filtering Systems

The reality is ….. your colon is like a coffee filter!
Many people believe that the pure water they drink goes straight from the stomach into the body. **Not true! Instead, that water is stored in your colon, and when the body requires more water, it withdraws it from the colon.**
This means that the colon wall is like the filter in a coffee maker. Any contaminants on the colon wall, like the coffee grounds, adds that substance to the water as it passes through (Figure 1.)

How contamination happens
Protein from hamburgers, eggs, chicken, etc. promotes adhesion of feces to the colon walls. Protein by nature is sticky. Look in any encyclopedia or online and you will find that the **first generation of glue** was processed from animals and fish. We are all familiar with the glue-like properties of protein laden feces on porcelain toilet bowls. Without a sufficient amount of fiber to clean the colon and absorb contaminants, as well as move them quickly through the colon, a residue builds up. The contaminating residue on colon walls that hasn't been eliminated remains in a stagnant, rotting state over the years. **The problem is, 90% of the water used by your body is filtered through the rotting residue on the colon**

walls. This really gives new meaning to the old saying, *"I feel shitty today."*

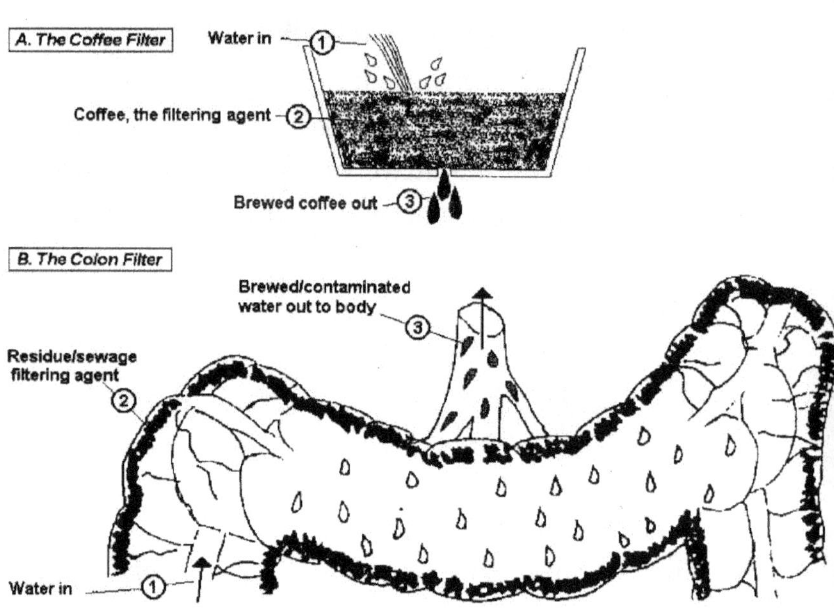

Figure 1: Shows water that is bi-directional going through the residue on the colon wall: A. Filters your water supply through rotting residue. B. Residue blocks waste from entering the colon from other organs.

BI-DIRECTIONAL, THE BIG SURPRISE

The blood vessels surrounding your colon that take moisture away are also bi- directional, meaning that they bring waste products from other body organs. If the colon wall contains rotting, stagnating contaminants, the waste cannot penetrate into the colon for elimination. Where does it go if it can't get through?

It's categorized according to what the waste is, then sent to its warehouse in the body (e.g., fats are sent to arterial walls, where it's called cholesterol, or it may be sent to the gallbladder and stored as gallstones or how about the minerals in waste stored in joints, which restricts movement and causes pain (arthritis)? [End Notes 7]

What else is contamination your water supply?

Check out any label at the supermarket. Here are a few from a label that we may consume on a weekly basis. How about propylene glycol, thiamine mononitrate or maltodextrin?

What does this stuff do that's being filtered into our water supply? It sounds like it should be found under a sink or at a gas station, not determining how we feel the next day or what health condition it is going to cause in the future.

But where are the other chemicals stored?

You know the ones on food labels that we can't pronounce. They can't get through into the colon either. Perhaps they're stored in the brain, where they cause anxiety, depression or just another sleepless night? Or maybe the latest chemical food additive is stored in **breast tissues.**

7- Water and Fiber

When drinking water, many of us are unaware of where it goes or what it does. In fact we find drinking water in many cases a huge inconvenience. In my case, I would stand at the kitchen sink, fill a glass up, take several swallows, fill again and call that two glasses of water. If I had a busy day planned, I would cut my water intake; because finding a bathroom became a real nuisance, thank God for fast food restaurants.

> **Hint:** If you have to go out and don't want this hassle, consume a bran muffin to absorb and entrain the water.

Two types of water

Free water is too much water (more than 16 ounces), consumed too quickly and at the wrong time. Because it's not mixed with fibrous food, the majority is absorbed by the small intestine and exits rapidly. We have all experienced two quick glasses (16 ounces) of water on an empty stomach. In a nutshell, it never reaches its intended destination, the colon.

Entrained water is a part of food. An example would be

the water that's part of an orange, cucumber or an apple.

Another example is dry cereal, which has the ability to absorb and retain water in its cellular structure, similar to a paper towel.

EXAMPLES OF FREE AND ENTRAINED WATER

The heavy rain storm with a large run off, flooding roads and basements (free water) compared to the soft soaking rain, absorbed by the soil (entrained water.)

Enlightening water facts

We are aware of how critical water is and the importance of the proper amounts. However, there are other factors in our water intake.

Evaporation can be very significant. The average body has approximately 15 square feet of area, or the size of a small kitchen found in an apartment. Consider how fast two glasses of water will disappear if evenly distributed over a flat surface. I've tried its 20 minutes – even faster outdoors in the sun.

Diuretics, such as coffee and soda, will greatly increase urination. In my case, I always thought that my consumption of 4 cups of coffee and 3 glasses of soda would count for water. Instead it depletes the body's water supply and increases urination per day of more than 1 quart.

Alcohol tends to evaporate our water supply too. Along with certain drugs.

The bottom line

You need the equivalent of 8 to 12 glasses of water per day (1 glass = 8 ounces) or approximately 64 to 96 swallows (1 swallow = 1 ounce) to meet normal water requirements. A medium-sized apple or orange is about 4 to 6 ounces of entrained water. A bowl of cereal about 4 ounces, if milk is used.

INSOLUBLE FIBER, TRAINING EQUIPMENT FOR THE COLON™

Just as a lineman uses weight training to achieve strength and a runner must increase mileage to build endurance, your colon needs training. The training equipment for this purpose is <u>insoluble fiber</u>. Like all training equipment, insoluble fiber must be used correctly for you to gain the benefits.

Insoluble fiber doesn't dissolve and adds bulk to your waste. It will absorb a large percentage of the water you consume, which achieves the expansion needed and softening of the feces. Soluble fiber from fruits and vegetables also expands the colon by producing water-absorbing bacteria and feces-moving gas. However, fruits and vegetables are digested in the small intestine and most do not appear in the stool as fiber.

Cabbage, for example, virtually disappears, but had a considerable effect on fecal output by 69% (Cummings et al., 1978a). [End Notes 8] **The problem with soluble fiber it's not consistent on a daily basis.**

Soluble fiber and carbon dioxide (gas is good)

Fruits and vegetables bring yeast (single-cell fungi) into the colon, and sugar starts the fermentation process. This process produces three types of gases: carbon dioxide, hydrogen and methane. For our purposes we shall only explore carbon dioxide.

Carbon dioxide is best known as the bubbly ingredient found in soda, beer, sparkling wines. Carbon dioxide provides an excellent shield or blanket to prevent oxidation. It is so efficient as an antioxidant that it is used in **industries** to process and package many foods, such as cheese, meats and eggs, to preserve their flavor and quality. [End Notes 9]

Insoluble fiber: What it is and how it works – from the experts

Insoluble fiber is found in the outside layer of the grains, corn and beans. It is generally removed in the manufacturing process in favor of product taste and profitability. But can still be obtained from cereal, whole wheat breads or beans. You have heard it described as **bran, roughage** and **cellulose.**

They do not dissolve in the small intestine the way fruit and vegetable fiber does. Bran, roughage and cellulose increase bulk by absorbing water, which expands feces to increase flowability.

Dimock (1937) stated ". . . the fiber of green vegetables and ordinary foodstuffs is more readily broken down in the alimentary tract (mouth to rectum) than that of wheat bran." This observation explains why the addition of fruits and vegetables to the diet so often **fails to prevent constipation**.

Hence, a diet may seem at first glance adequate enough in fiber to produce satisfactory bowel habits, but may be lacking in insoluble fiber. [End Notes 10]

How insoluble fiber works

A good example of how insoluble fiber functions is the paper towel, which contains filaments that trap (entrain) water, expands like a sponge, and then becomes very pliable.

Insoluble fiber expands the colon by absorbing large amounts of water and increasing feces volume, which makes the repetitions of the peristaltic contractions (colon pump) two to three times more effective, so the feces moves two to three times faster.

Insoluble fiber also cleans the colon by absorbing contaminants (the stuff on food labels you can't pronounce) so that <u>they are eliminated instead of being absorbed into the blood stream</u>. In addition, insoluble fiber increases flowability by softening and bulking the feces so they can readily negotiate the colon's 90-, 180-, 270-, and 360-degree turns and obstructions.

Finally, the bulk/volume of the feces due to fiber content sends the correct signals to your central nervous system when it is time to eliminate.

How fiber works in your colon

The cereal label in Figure 2 shows that the cereal contains 9 grams of insoluble fiber per ½ cup (about two handfuls.)

Nutrition Facts

Serving Size   1/2 Cup (31 g/1.1 oz.)
Servings per Package

Amount Per Serving	Cereal	
Calories	80	120
Calories from Fat	10	10
	% Daily Value**	
Total Fat 1g*	2%	2%
Saturated Fat 0g	0%	0%
Cholesterol 0mg	0%	0%
Sodium 80mg	3%	6%
Potassium 350mg	10%	16%
Total Carbohydrate 23g	8%	10%
Dietary Fiber 10g	40%	40%
Soluble Fiber 1g		
Insoluble Fiber 9g		
Other Carbohydrate 7g		
Protein 4g		

Figure 2: Cereal label showing nutrition facts, including amount of fiber.

For our example,(illustration continues on page 42,) we are going to use two full cups of cereal, (4 servings), so we have a total of 40 grams of fiber. We will forget about the 4 grams of soluble fiber (shown as round bubbles in

Figure 3), because it is inconsistent in increasing feces volume and producing feces-moving gas.

This leaves us with 36 grams of insoluble fiber (shown as half- rectangles in Figure 3.) When combined with an adequate amount of water, this insoluble fiber bulks the feces so that it moves almost halfway through the colon as shown in Figure 3. This is what we want to happen. Next, we'll contrast that with the opposite – a diet of inadequate fiber.

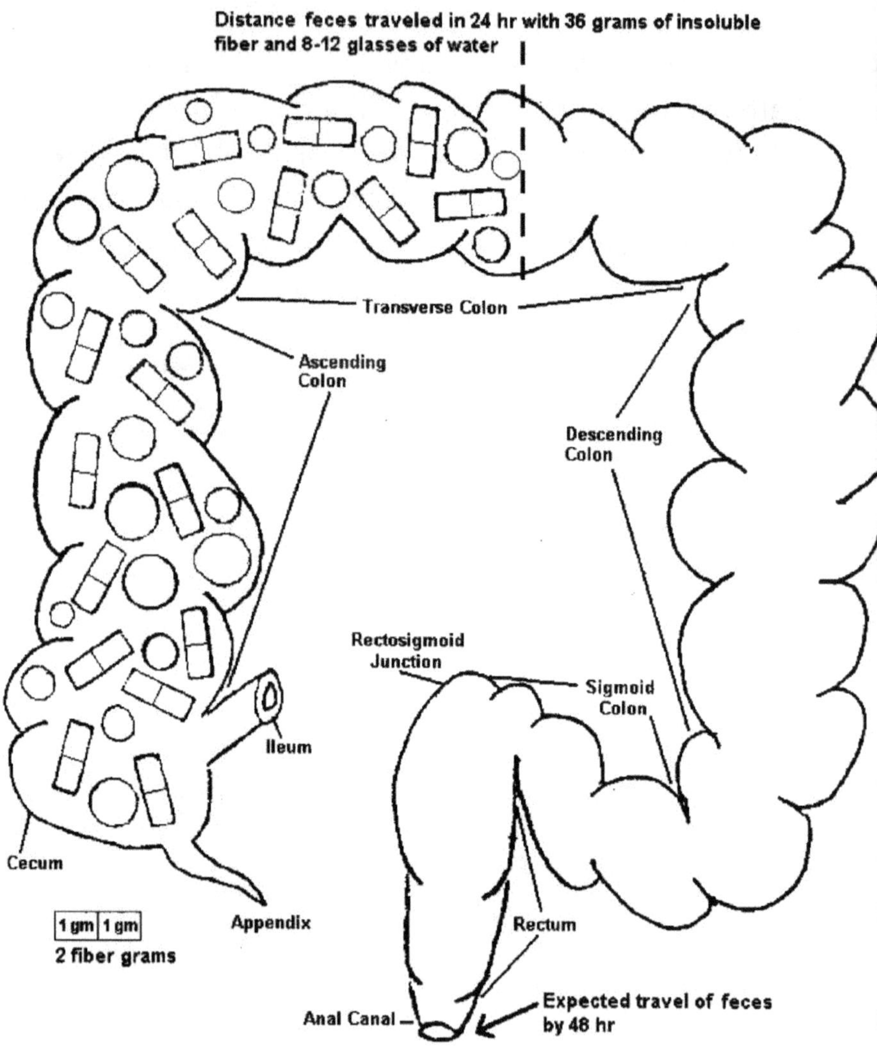

Figure 3: Example of a healthy colon, half full, after eating. The colon sides are clean of residue, absorbed by insoluble fiber (rectangles.) Soluble fibers (circles) are ignored due to inconsistency. Transit time may vary depending on size, shape, and condition of the colon.

Important: The colon shown on the previous page, is a
textbook colon. Yours may look like a tangled
extension cord (see Figure 11, page 75) and it may
be impacting other organs.

How the lack of fiber affects your colon

Protein-laden feces are two to three times smaller in
volume, but weigh about the same as a high-fiber stool,
because they lack sufficient insoluble fiber to absorb water.
They travel only one third as far in a given time period as
a high-fiber stool, so they take two to three times longer to
eliminate, which is dangerous.

Protein and fats lack the ability to absorb/entrain water
therefore they don't expand like fiber does. Did you ever
try to combine water with oil or wash grease off plates with
water? Protein, high in residue (glue-like qualities) adheres
to the colon wall, rots and stagnates, then water filters
through this sludge bringing the contaminates to your
blood stream.

(The paragraph above is so important, please re-read.)

The result of a low-fiber diet is shown in Figure 4, which is
an unhealthy colon.

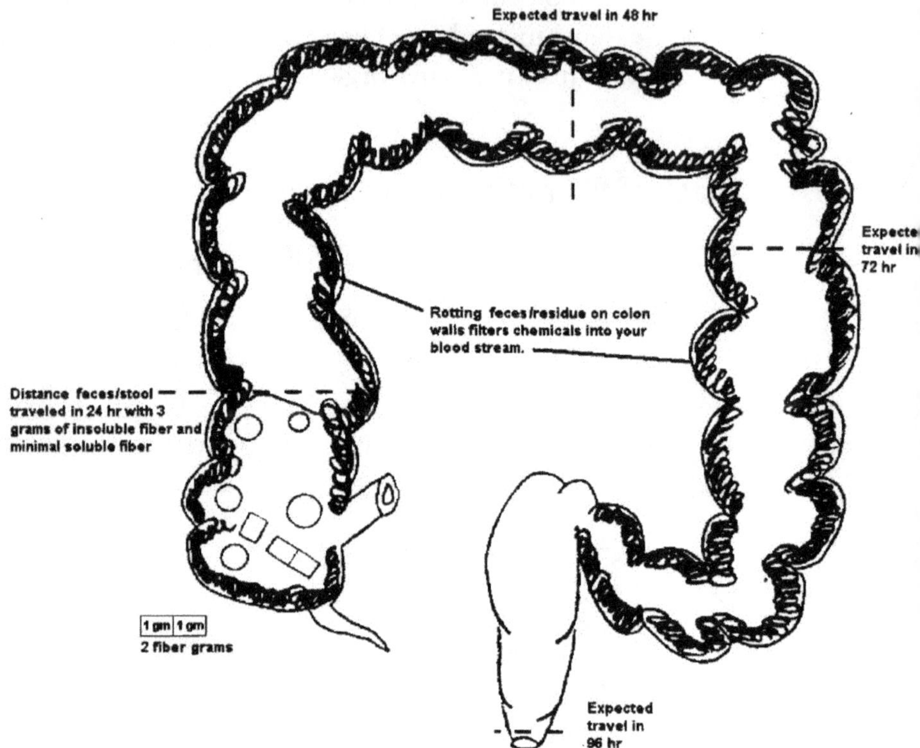

Figure 4: The colon wall, coated with residue, combined with the slow movement of the feces, due to the lack of fiber and water, leads to an unhealthy colon. Movement of the feces is two to three times slower, therefore filtering water through the colon lining, bringing toxic waste into your blood stream.

8- How Protein, Carbohydrates, Fats, and Starches Work in the Colon

Protein

In the body
It's important for growth, development, and energy. Protein creates hormones, enzymes, and tissues. However, our diet of meat, fish, and dairy products **approaches 5 to 6 times** more than the 50 to 60 grams needed per day. (Half a steak is approximately between 50 – 60 grams.) With this much protein, we are really trying to glue our colon together.

It's the stuff of glue
The Webster's Dictionary definition of glue: "(1) A hard protein gelatin obtained by boiling skins, hooves, and other animal substances in water and used as a strong adhesive; (2) any of various preparations of this or a similar substance used as an adhesive."
We have all experienced the glue-like qualities of feces and the need for the powerful cleaners sold for cleaning toilet bowls.

Is the colon trying to glue it together
Protein slows the process because it's sticky, slow-moving, high in residue, and adheres to the colon wall like eggs on a plate. Protein provides less than one third the volume of fiber to bulk, expand and clean the colon, which means

your protein meal will take up to 3 times longer to reach the anal canal.

Why?

Protein will absorb/entrain only 20% of its weight in moisture, whereas insoluble fiber may absorb up to 400% of its weight in moisture to expand the feces. Commercial fiber, **psyllium seed husks** will absorb 3000% of its weight, with a super high grade, up to 55x its weight or 5500%.

What about fat, carbohydrates and starches?

Fat

Webster's definition of fat: "an oily material found in animal tissue." Fat is also found in dairy items, such as whole milk, cream and cheese. It is high in residue, slows transit time and will not absorb water.

Simple carbohydrates

These are sugars from fruits such as apples, oranges, and grapefruit. They are considered unrefined sugars, while desserts, candy bars, and table sugar contain refined and processed sugars. Choose fruits for soluble fiber and their fermentation (i.e., carbon dioxide) value, which helps the colon pump move the stool.

Complex carbohydrates

These come from vegetables, whole grains, and beans. They provide both soluble fiber and insoluble fiber. How much insoluble fiber you actually consume depends on the manufacturing process (see the wheat grain on page 50.)

Starches

Starch is a white, tasteless solid found in rice, corn, wheat, beans and other vegetables (complex carbohydrates.) Starches are manipulated during the manufacturing process to achieve maximum productivity and profit. It is the same stuff used in industry to add rigidity or stiffen a product (i.e., garments.) Breads, doughnuts and crackers provide an abundance of starch, which leads to stool stiffness.

9- The Colon Pump

Going the distance in 48 hours
To meet this goal, the feces must negotiate the colon, **a free floating organ**, with many different turns, ranging from 90 to 360 degrees. It may deviate from its basic horseshoe configuration to one that looks like a tangled extension cord, with many different turns and diameters, but nevertheless winds up in the same place.
(See Figure 11, page 75)

SO WHAT MOVES THIS STUFF?

The first method: *The most efficient method is repetitive peristaltic contractions. To simulate this action, take a really ripe banana (one with brown spots), and squeeze in your hand by applying pressure one finger at a time until the banana basically squirts out of your grasp. This type of action is repeated again and again in the colon until elimination occurs. The really ripe banana in our body is the high- volume, moisture-laden, high-fiber stool. Conversely, a flat, out-of-shape colon loaded with protein (glue) just isn't efficient. Try to imagine a semi-flat sewer pipe, water pipe or drain, trying to move something with the consistency of mud!*

The second method: *The second method is the assist from gas, manufactured by soluble fiber, which creates pressure from behind and through the feces. It may:*

- *Gently help the contractions move the feces*
- *Create a mass movement, with the entire amount of feces moving suddenly towards the rectum when the pressure behind feces (gas) is greater than that in the front. We have all experienced that sudden urge at a very inopportune time.*
- *Create extreme pain, which in most cases may be nothing more than gas expanding the colon wall because it is trapped behind feces laden with protein and starch that lack the correct moisture and fiber content to move.*
- ***Both methods are needed for maximum efficiency.***

10- The Wheat Grain

The cornerstone of health, it's this simple.

Understanding what happened

A lot of us have visited an historic site, where a guide would make the comment, "This was the old mill, the farmers brought their grain here to mill and make flour, so that mom could make cookies and pies."

But this was before the industrial revolution, when the old mill couldn't separate the starch from the bran and we had to use the whole grain.

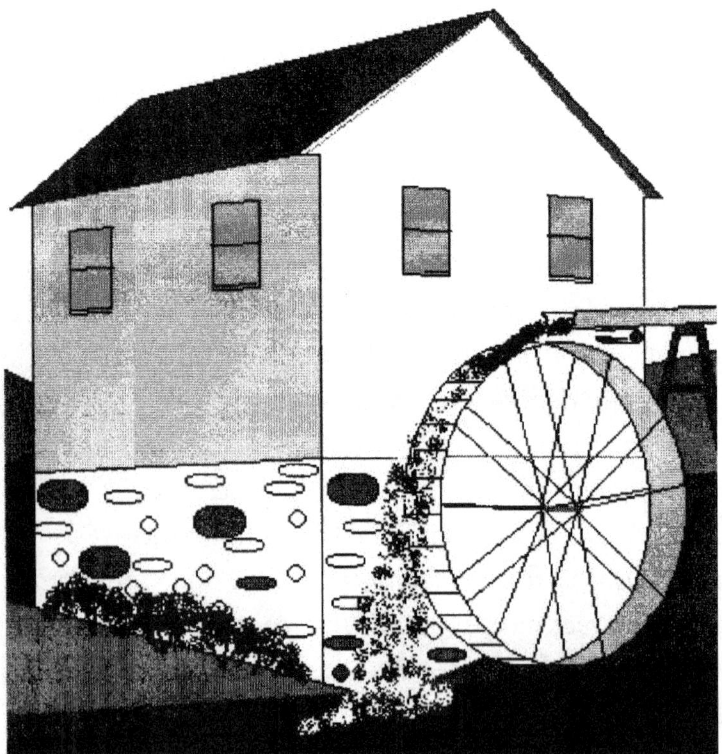

Figure 5: The old mill

But now

Our grain is now manipulated, separated and controlled to suit products, enhance taste, and increase product profitability. The bran is disposed of, so unfortunately now the consumer is paying the price with exploding health issues in every part of the body.

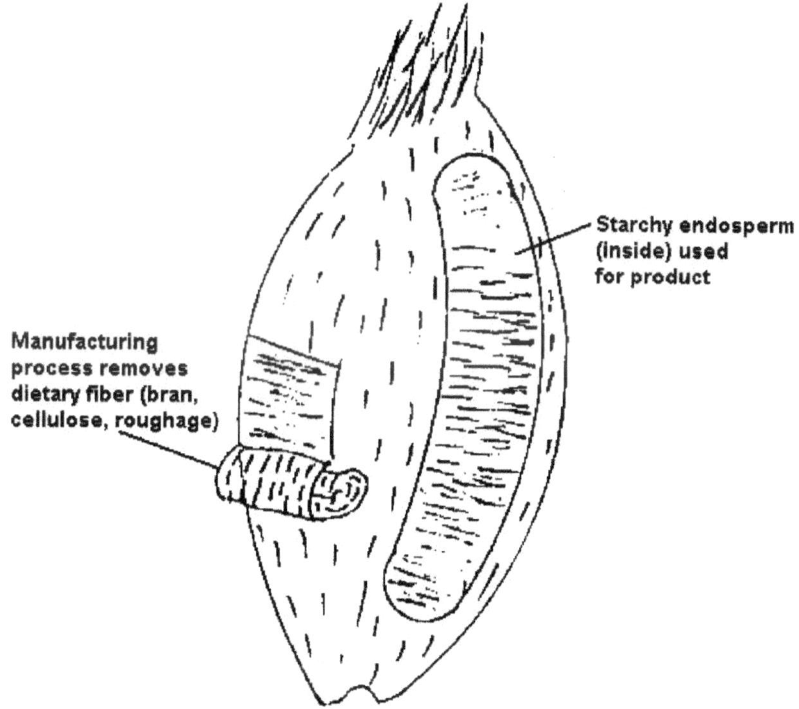

Figure 6: The wheat grain, magnified 100 times.

Your health – now just floor sweepings

The bran that is removed from wheat grains is now located in a barrel at your local health food store. It is called "miller's bran," looks a lot like sawdust and sells for about two dollars a pound. **It just may be the healthiest product in the store.**

11- The Solution

The shopping routine

First, it's into a large supermarket, awash in bright colors and music all choreographed to maximize profit and emphasize health. Once through the front door, the programmed path leads the consumer through the fresh fruits and vegetables, which paint the picture of health for sale. We can't miss here. Just pick any fruit or vegetable. They're all mostly soluble fiber.

What's next?

The following aisles are decorated, color-coordinated with product brands, designed by artists. The artwork on packaging appeals to your senses. It's museum quality and it's intended to distract you from reading the labels. For example, that box of crackers with pleasing natural scenery alluding to health, in fact has **minimal fiber**, and mostly profitable starch.

The fact is

The typical box of cereal with all its attractive "natural" scenery actually contains a product with 1 gram or less of insoluble dietary fiber. In comparison, if we were buying a new car, one of the first figures we would look at is **miles per gallon**. If it's really low, we won't even consider that car because it affects our economic health. When buying snacks, cereals or breads, try thinking about maybe **inches**

per hour in the colon, which affects both our physical health and our economic health.

The most important aisle: Cereal (insoluble fiber)

It's located in the middle of the store, it's the most colorful, with cartoon characters and animals dominating the place. All the kids are gleefully pointing out to Mom what to buy. It's all there at their eye level, except any cereal containing more than 3 grams of fiber. High-fiber cereals are up on the highest shelf, out of reach and almost out of sight.

What are we looking for here? It's easy, any cereal with 7 grams or more of insoluble fiber per ¾ cup. If we consume 1½ cups, we're already at 14 grams for the day, and have the option to add 1 to 2 tablespoons of miller's bran for another 2-5 grams for 19 grams.

Nutrition Facts

Serving Size: 3/4 cup (30g)
Servings per Package: About 12

Amount Per Serving

Calories 90	Calories from Fat 10

	% Daily Value**
Total Fat 1g*	2%
Saturated Fat 0g	0%
Cholesterol 0mg	0%
Sodium 70 mg	3%
Potassium 120mg	3%
Total Carbohydrate 24g	8%
(Dietary Fiber 8g)	32%
Soluble Fiber 1g	
Insoluble Fiber 7g	
Sugars 6g	
Protein 3g	

Figure 7: Nutrition label from high-fiber cereal product.

Lunch, dinner or a snack will add another 5 to 10 grams. Also, include one or two teaspoons of psyllium seed husks, depending on your requirements, in the afternoon and eat what you want, within reason. (See pages 46 & 96, psyllium seed husks)

Breakfast for kids???

This is where it starts.

The bright and colorful animated box of cereal, sold for your **child's amusement**, has 2 grams of insoluble dietary fiber, and enough sugar to ruin your day. With a serving size of ¾ cup, your child will need the whole box and more for his daily insoluble fiber requirements.

Nutrition Facts		
Serving Size	3/4 cup (31 g/1.1 oz.)	
Servings per Package		About 14
Amount Per Serving	Cereal	
Calories	120	160
Calories from Fat	0	0
	% Daily Value**	
Total Fat 0g*	0%	0%
Saturated Fat 0g	0%	0%
Cholesterol 0mg	0%	0%
Sodium 150mg	6%	9%
Potassium 20mg	1%	6%
Total Carbohydrate 28g	9%	11%
Dietary Fiber 2g	3%	3%
Sugars 12g		
Other Carbohydrate 15g		

Figure 8: Nutrition label from low-fiber kid's cereal.

Helpful options: Save the colorful box to hold your homemade fiber mix.

Proof is in the shopping cart

Match the contents to the shopper. Check out the cart loaded with brightly colored, low-fiber items. You'll usually find a shopper who is overweight, looks tired, and is lacking in energy. More than likely the person also has health problems. Check the cart with fruits and vegetables, for bean products and high dietary fiber cereals. No mystery here, the shopper looks good and has energy.

Breakfast is the most important meal

It's an old saying, but with a different meaning. Ask 100 people, and they will generally say "breakfast gives me energy for the day," but they should say "breakfast gives me the best opportunity to consume insoluble fiber for the day."

12-Getting Started One Way or Another

Remember this: Protein sticks and slows, water flows. Insoluble fiber bulks and softens. Soluble fiber ferments and explodes (in a good way.)

You have a choice
The goal is to start reducing transit time towards 48 hours, you may decide to clean your colon or you may just increase your fiber intake and let nature take its course.

If you choose to clean your colon.
Finish reading this book, and make a decision based upon the information. Directions for bowel cleansing can be found in the instructions of Fleet Phospho-Soda, which is often used in medical procedures. I asked this question to the colorectal specialist who did up to 30 colonoscopies per week. "How clean does your colon become when doing the bowel cleaning?" His answer "so clean I can see the small blood vessels in the colon wall." He also mentioned that an enema is of no use for cleaning.

Check for constipation/water and fiber
Count the glasses of water or liquid that you consume per day; be aware of the caffeinated/alcoholic beverages that take moisture away, by causing excessive urination. Water intake must be a minimum 8 glasses per day or the equivalent every day. **Please remember: if you are not**

**used to water, it may take weeks or longer just to bring
your water level to normal (i.e., to rehydrate all organs.)**
Count your insoluble fiber grams, just use the label on the
box and check out serving size. While dining out, count
white breads, doughnuts and pastry as 0 grams. A bowl of
bean soup as 7 grams, pizza as 1 gram per slice, hamburger
and hotdog rolls as 0 grams (some may contain higher),
eight pretzels as 2 grams (who stops at eight pretzels?), or
20 potato chips as 1 gram. The number has to be a
minimum 25-35 grams insoluble fiber per day, every day.

It's so simple. Soluble fiber creates the driving force.
Apples, prunes and cabbage are the best for creating
fermentation.
They're moisture grabbing, carbon dioxide gas producing,
bacteria multipliers that are easy to use. All fruits and
vegetables bring their own special something to the party.
Don't forget those healthy leftovers in the refrigerator,
they react real fast because of the large good bacteria count
gathered in storage.
The minimum is at least an apple and a salad every day.

THE HARDEST PART OF THIS IS...

*The challenging part, in the beginning, is that everything
takes place 24 to 48 hours later, which in my case was
difficult. Why? If you're feeling good today, you're not
concerned about those great tasting, zero-fiber jelly doughnuts
for breakfast or the hamburger and fries for lunch and dinner.*

The next check

In the next couple of days, play close attention to the signs of constipation/rotting residue on the colon wall. These include constant tiredness, lack of strength, strong smelling urine, indigestion, heartburn, bad breath, a coated tongue, strong smelling feces, strong foot odor, and straining to eliminate.

Not knowing what is normal, we may have always reached for pain relief pills, antacid tablets, vitamins, or a laxative to correct these conditions.

Checking out our current transit time

This simple check measures the time food takes for the trip through the entire system, from intake (mouth) to exit (anus.) There are easy ways to accomplish this.

The outside of a corn kernel will not dissolve in the small intestine and will make the entire trip. It's easily spotted as specks of yellow in the stool. **Try a serving of canned corn.** Peanuts also work, as long as you are not allergic to them; chew and swallow two handfuls (not too many; they can cause constipation.) They will show up in the stool or on toilet paper.

The corn and peanuts show up slowly, a little bit at first and then more, followed by the remainder over the next day or two, which is normal. Don't worry if you have a straggler or two a week later.

Checking out our stool

The color, shape, consistency and size of our stools give us information on our condition.

The small round stool

The small, rounded stool, which resembles rabbit pellets ½ to ¾ inches in diameter, is a highly constipated condition, later resulting in the use of laxatives.

- One movement or less per day, consists of a few or many pellets.

- Requires straining for 10 to 15 minutes to produce (condition causes hemorrhoids)

- Dark brown, almost black in color (dried out)

- Offensive odor

- Contains too much protein (daily requirement needed only 50-60 grams, about as much as half a small apple)

- Contains less than 60% moisture (less than 4 glasses of water per day)

- Contains a small amount of insoluble fiber (2 to 3 grams)

- Contains a small amount of soluble fiber (1 fruit or a vegetable.)

- **Transit time is an unhealthy 96 hours or more**

The 3" to 6" long, packed-together stool

Some may consider this a normal stool; it resembles small ½ to ¾ inch diameter ovals packed together. It is a constipated condition (see Figure 12.)

- One movement or less per day

- Requires 5 to 10 minutes of straining to produce

- Dark brown in color

- May or may not have offensive odor

- Contains a large amount of protein

- Contains 60 to 65% moisture (less than six glasses of water per day)

- Contains a small amount of insoluble fiber (3 to 5 grams)

- May contain acceptable amounts of soluble fiber (two fruits and two vegetables per day)

- **Transit time an unhealthy 72 hours or more**

The 6" to 12" or longer softer stool

This stool is softer, smooth in appearance, like being squeezed from a tube – a large step towards health.

- One large movement or more per day

- Requires less than 5 minutes to produce

- Lighter brown in color, reflecting more

moisture and fiber content

- Bran specks start to appear in the toilet bowel (insoluble fiber)

- Correct amount of protein for body requirements

- Contains 70 to 80% moisture (equivalent of 8 glasses of water per day)

- Contains minimum daily insoluble fiber requirements (25 grams)

- Contains soluble fiber in line with body requirements (2 fruits, 2 vegetables)

- **Transit time approaching target of 48 hours**

The loose ragged stool, longer than 12", twice per day

This type of stool is the ultimate, what we're striving for on a daily basis.

- Two or more movements per day

- Produced in less than a minute or two

- Light brown in color, reflecting moisture, fiber content and transit time.

- Contains 80 to 85% moisture (equivalent to 8

to 12 glasses of water per day)

- Contains maximum daily insoluble fiber requirements (25 to 35 grams)

- Contains soluble fiber mixture that works for you (enough gas to move feces quickly through colon)

- **Transit time under 48 hours**

Stool volume will increase 2 to 3 times because of additional fiber and moisture content.

The too loose, liquid type, high frequency stool

This type of stool reflects too much liquid, soluble and insoluble fiber. If however, excess fiber and moisture are not present and the condition persists it may be attributed to an irritation in the colon, causing the colon to react, trying to rid itself of the irritation, which is called chronic diarrhea. Fiber may correct this by absorbing the irritant, expanding the colon, then eliminating it. (This is described on page 26.)

1. Stool volume will increase two to three times on fiber, so you should allow sufficient time to empty the sigmoid colon as well as the descending colon.

2. Each colon is different depending on size, shape and configuration (see page 75.) It may even have a 360-degree turn in the descending colon, so you must set aside up to 15 minutes of stool time, twice per day.

3. The urge to stool, because of correct fiber and moisture content, may now be just a full feeling in the lower stomach rather than the emergency urge we are accustomed to.

13-The Weight Loss Connection

Insoluble fiber helps with weight loss in three ways.

First

The insoluble fiber you consume passes through your system, it is not absorbed.   If you consume 30 grams per day, 365 days x 30 grams = 10,950 grams per year. At 450 grams to the pound, the weight savings to you   per year could be 24.3 pounds.

Second

Insoluble fiber may absorb up to 400% of its weight in water, thus creating 2 to 3 times the feces volume of protein, leading to a fuller feeling, which reduces the need to snack or overeat. Why? Because the transverse colon passes under the stomach, so if it's expanded by fiber, it pushes into the stomach, creating a fuller feeling.

Third

Insoluble fiber blocks fat-absorbing enzymes by **"tying them up,"** thus decreasing the amount of fat that can be absorbed. [End Notes 11]

The easy stretch to being overweight.

Companies are removing fiber from our foods. To achieve the full feeling that fiber supplies our bodies, we eat 2 to 3 times more food (protein, fat and starch) to compensate, which may explain overeating and obesity.

Could it be just this simple???

Please realize that the average food intake per day is 2 pounds. Less than 10 percent of the food you consume makes the entire trip through your system because 90 percent is absorbed by the body. The remaining 10 percent is expanded by two to three times in weight and volume by the correct fiber, water and bacteria content. That volume increases the number of movements per day and increases stool transit time by 2 to 3 times.

14-Starting Fiber Consumption Cautiously

Internal exercise

If your fiber intake is low, with the intake of soluble fiber less than a fruit and/or a vegetable per day and insoluble fiber less than 2 grams, **then it is extremely important to proceed slowly.** Just like you would in a successful exercise program for other body parts.

Why? Because the addition of too much water-holding fiber expands too rapidly for your out of shape, flabby, unexercised colon. In short, your colon can't take all that exercise at once. Over the years it has remained almost flat, corroded and stagnating (Figure 9,) instead of being toned, clean and round (Figure 10.)

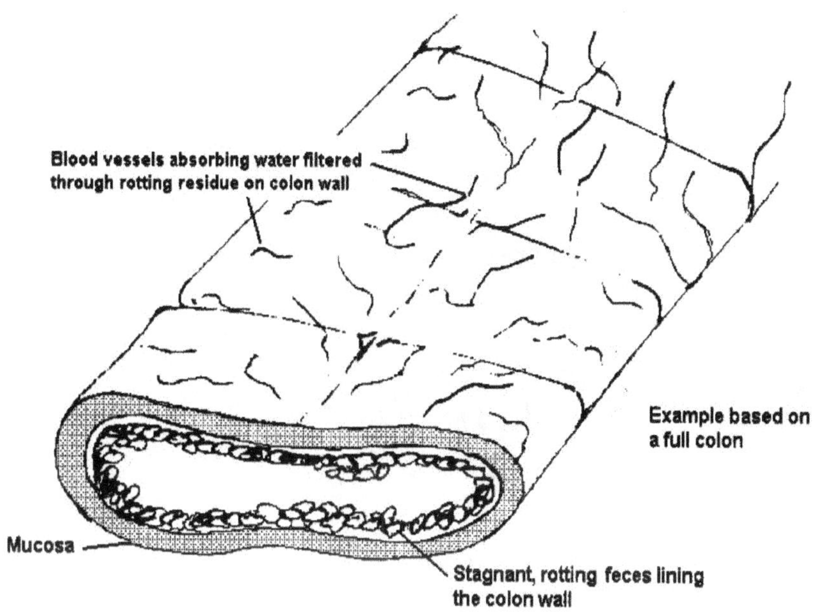

Figure 9: Inside the out-of-shape colon or "This is your colon on too much protein/fat/starch" (Example based on a *full colon*, which still remains flat from lack of fiber.)

Figure 9, shows how the sagging, collapsed colon is lined with residue through which water is filtered on the way to your blood stream. This illustration also gives insight into the effect of a high-protein diet, which can't bulk the colon as insoluble fiber does. Pumping (contractions) are not efficient, feces dry faster, and the time required for elimination is 4-5 days.

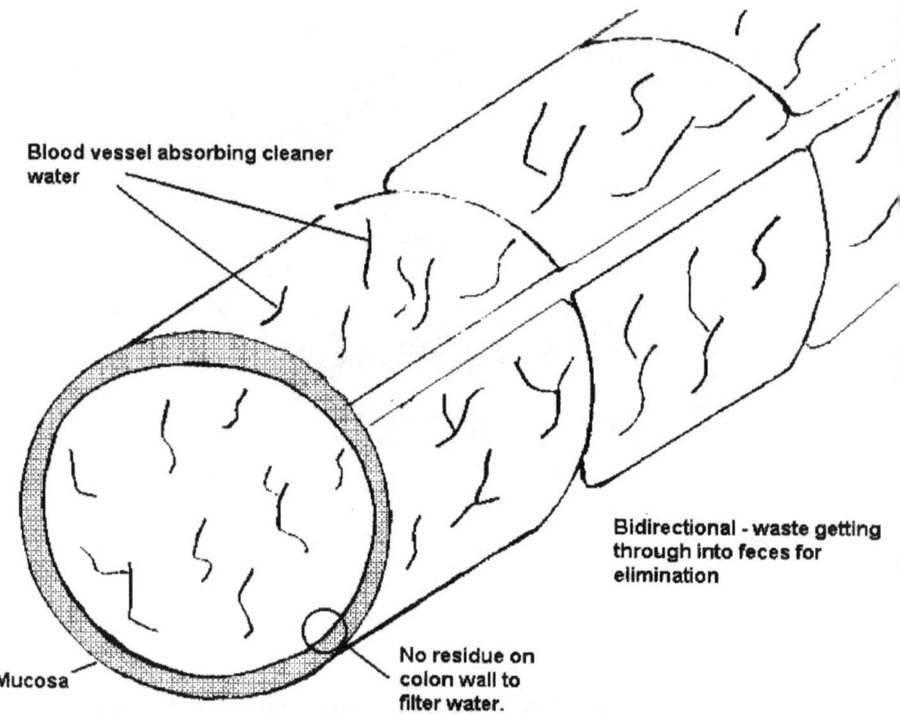

Figure 10: Inside the in-shape colon or "This is your colon on insoluble fiber." (Example based on a full colon.)

In contrast to Figure 9, Figure 10 shows that a healthy, round colon is clean so that water absorbed into your body is not contaminated. This illustration gives insight into the benefits of high fiber intake, which bulks and cleans the colon, makes contractions (pumping action) efficient, and reduces elimination time to less than 48 hours.

The result of too much too soon

- Insoluble fiber will try to expand the out of shape colon, but failing to, it just clogs and blocks the colon. This may make you doubt the value of fiber and discontinue its use.

- Soluble fiber may create too much gas and expand the colon causing gas pains by trying to expand the **out of shape colon** (Figure 9.) Gas pains are simply 2 pounds of pressure on the colon wall caught behind a stool.

Starting with fiber (the training equipment)

Soluble fiber

Proceed slowly and try different ingredients. Fruits and veggies produce friendly bacteria and yeast. Consider commercial developed probiotics, which contain friendly bacteria in large amounts as a prime mover. Please remember everyone's chemistry is different and will respond differently to each ingredient. Here are a few ideas from my own experiences.

- Prunes are nature's laxative.

- Apples contain pectin, a prime mover. Remember to remove the skin which can cause constipation.

- Fermented foods and drinks are a great prime mover. They help the good bacteria grow in your gut: raw sauerkraut, kimchi and pickles, kombucha to name a few. (If pasteurized, it will kill the friendly bacteria.)

- Soups that combine different ingredients (e.g., onions, carrots, zucchini, and beans) work well.

- Bananas act as a prebiotic, giving the friendly bacteria a place to grow and flourish.

Insoluble fiber

Try **different cereals**. There are many types of fibers used in making cereal; check for high fiber content and variety.

Think about all those bright-colored field markers you've seen by the side of the road indicating various hybrid wheat and corn. Here are the others we may look for: wheat bran, ground oats, long grain brown rice, rye, corn bran, winter wheat, barley, and sesame seeds.

Remember, the more varieties of bran, the more effective. Most cereals have only wheat bran, which is found in less expensive cereals.

If you feel heavy, sluggish or tired from wheat products, you may be allergic to all of them or to a particular wheat product. It may be to your advantage to try other products.

How to train with fiber (equivalent of 8-12 glasses of liquid required)

Remember, each colon has a different size and shape, and is in a different condition and location, so results will vary.

Try this. Work toward your goal of producing one healthy stool per day, possible two over a period of three weeks to three months. The key is to keep your stomach comfortable through the process.

Week or month one

Increase soluble fiber by adding fruits and vegetables to your diet gradually.

Increase insoluble fiber slowly with a breakfast cereal. Make sure the cereal you choose has 7 grams or more of insoluble fiber. You can also add 1 to 2 teaspoons of miller's bran bought at a health food store.

In the afternoon or early evening, use a teaspoon of psyllium seed husks mixed in a glass of water or juice, at least 8 to 12oz. Continue your regular diet, if comfortable go to week or month two.

Week or month two

Increase soluble fiber to an apple, without the skin, plus a vegetable or bean soup and have a salad with dinner.

Increase insoluble fiber to 12 grams per day and use 2 to 3 teaspoons of miller's bran.

In the afternoon or early evening, use a teaspoon of psyllium seed husks in water or juice.

Check stools for color, shape, softness, using the descriptions on pages 61-64 to determine the stage you have reached. If you are comfortable, go on to week or month three.

Week or month three

Increase soluble fiber to one more fruit or vegetable. Increase insoluble fiber to 25-35 grams per day.

In the afternoon or early evening, use a teaspoon of psyllium seed husks. This will help curb your appetite before dinner.

> Experiment: For a complete understanding, put a teaspoon of psyllium seed husks in a ¼ cup of water and stir, let sit for 20 minutes.

Check again on pages 61-64. Increase of decrease fiber as needed to achieve the results you want.

Remember, this is not a diet; it's what is needed to support your eating habits so you can remain healthy and decrease or stabilize your weight.

15-Elimination

– W. Thompson [End Notes 12]

Things to do today

Until now elimination just didn't rank high on our list of things to do. In fact, if it didn't bother us, once every three days was fine. Most wouldn't disagree, which may explain the lack of interest and consequences of not producing a stool at least once a day.

Remember the problem

It's the flowability of feces that enable them to negotiate the 90-, 180-, 270-, and 360-degree turns and go quickly through different colon diameters and configurations (Figure 11.)
Flowability is achieved by consuming the correct amounts of fiber and water.

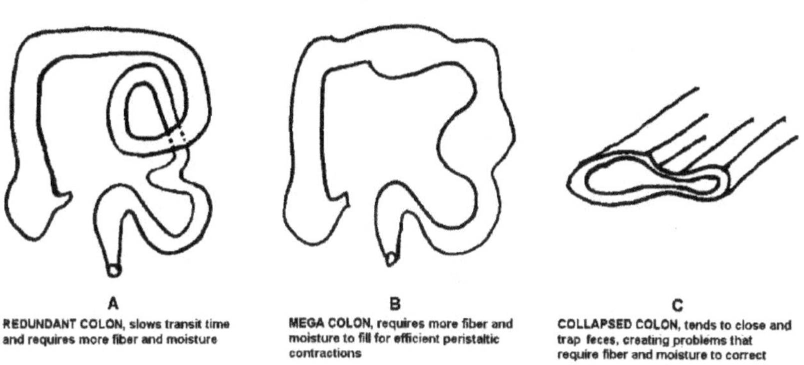

Figure 11: Different colon configurations. An individual may have one or a combination of all three types of colons.

What is yours – A, B, C – or worse?

Look at the colons shown in Figure 11. Finding out which one you have just might be your key to health. Most people are convinced that the recommended standard colonoscopy is enough to check for problems. However, a colonoscopy is like going through a tunnel in the middle of a city. For planning, a roadmap with accurate sizes and exact locations may be needed. This roadmap is called a double-contrast barium enema or the newer virtual colonoscopy using CT scans. Either one would show the routing, size, and location of the colon. For more information consult page 94 in the Appendix of this book. (*Remember the colon is a free floating organ.*)

The rectosigmoid junction: Your colon's hairpin curve (Figure 13, page 80)

Before the sixties we were literally a stand-up society, spending more time in manufacturing and farming.

Commuting consisted of walking to our jobs and communicating meant getting out of a chair to carry a message to the next office or another floor. Now the opposite is true. We are a sit-down society.

Constipation has arrived.

Sitting has become the norm, it affects the rectosigmoid junction, which is basically an area that compresses through sitting, (Figure 13.) It is the most difficult turn in the colon.

Think of it this way

Your colon is a four-lane highway, which narrows into one lane with a hairpin turn at the end. Every day you take this highway to work and every day you forget the turn is there and every day, you never look at the gas and oil gauge (water and fiber in our case) and every day you run out of sufficient gas and oil at the curve.

What happens next

You get out of the car, and push and strain to get it on the shoulder of the road so it doesn't cause a huge traffic jam. Or worse yet, if it won't move, we call for help, a tow truck (i.e., a laxative.) How come in a car, if we forget gas and oil we never say, "my car is constipated or I have irritable car syndrome?"

The exercise connection

We have always been advised that exercise helps, but never knew all the reasons why. If we go for a walk, use the stairs, do any kind of exercise, or even vigorously move the abdomen, we are moving the colon, a free floating organ, around inside the abdominal cavity.

The garden hose

It's like moving the hose and watching water appear at one end. In our case, it may be just enough to straighten a colon curve or reconfigure it so the stool can pass through. The more physical movement the better.

Figures 12, 13, 14, (pages 79-81,) illustrates the important role of the rectosigmoid junction. Figure 12 shows how a low-moisture stool can block and Figure 13 shows how sitting makes the problem worse.

In contrast, Figure 14 shows how a high-fiber, high-moisture stool expands the colon and increases flowability to get around the obstruction. Houston valves hold the wet, high- fiber stool, which flows through the smallest opening and enlarges it. Straining is not needed to pass through the junction. (Keep in mind that this figure shows a "typical" junction; in fact, no two junctions are alike; each will have a different configuration.)

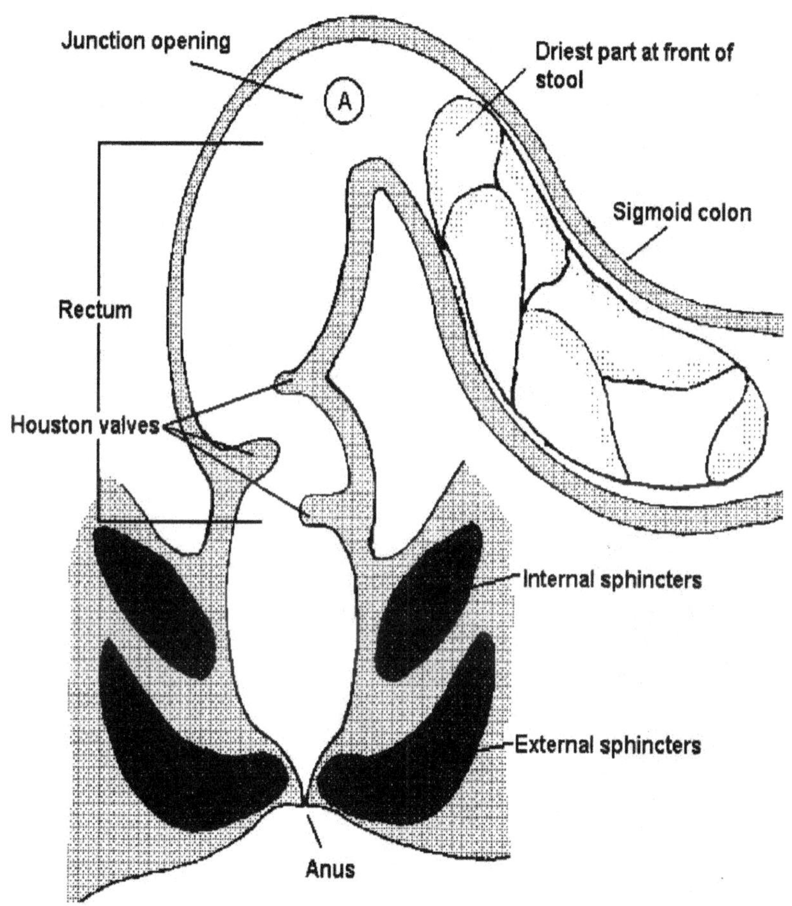

Figure 12: Rectosigmoid junction of a standing, active person with a high-protein, low-moisture stool. Straining may not drive this stool through the junction (A) without a laxative. Sleep or exercise may help relax this area.

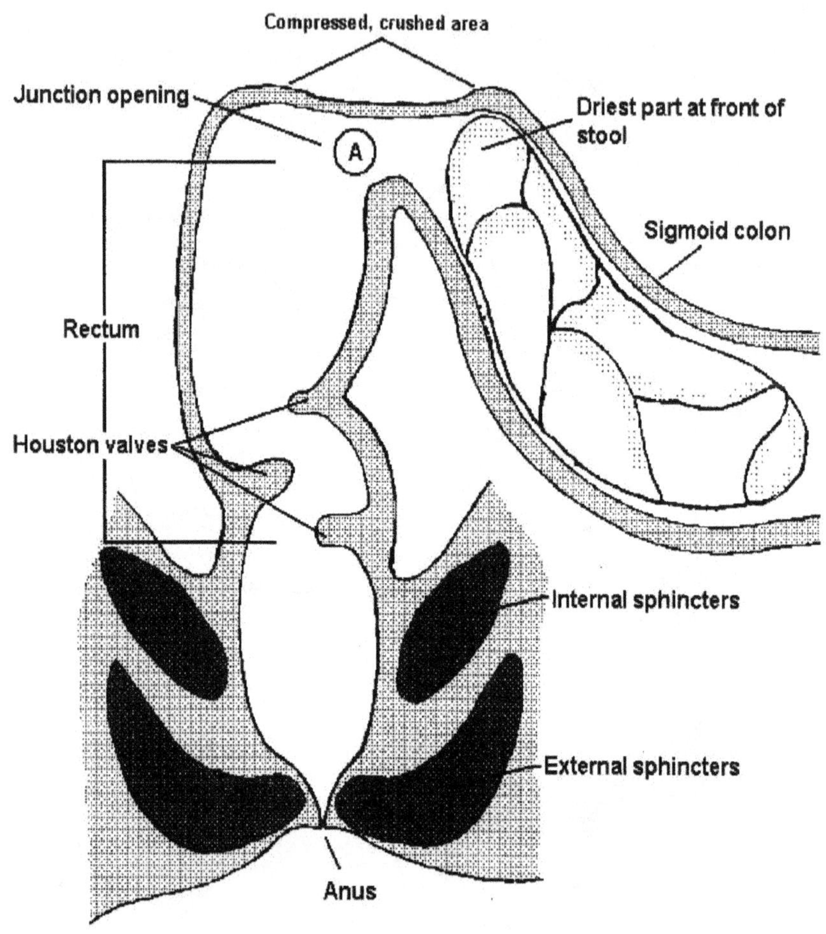

Figure 13: Rectosigmoid junction (compressed/ crushed area) of a sitting, commuting person with a high-protein, low-moisture stool. Straining may not drive this stool through the junction (A) without a laxative. Sleep or exercise may help relax this area.

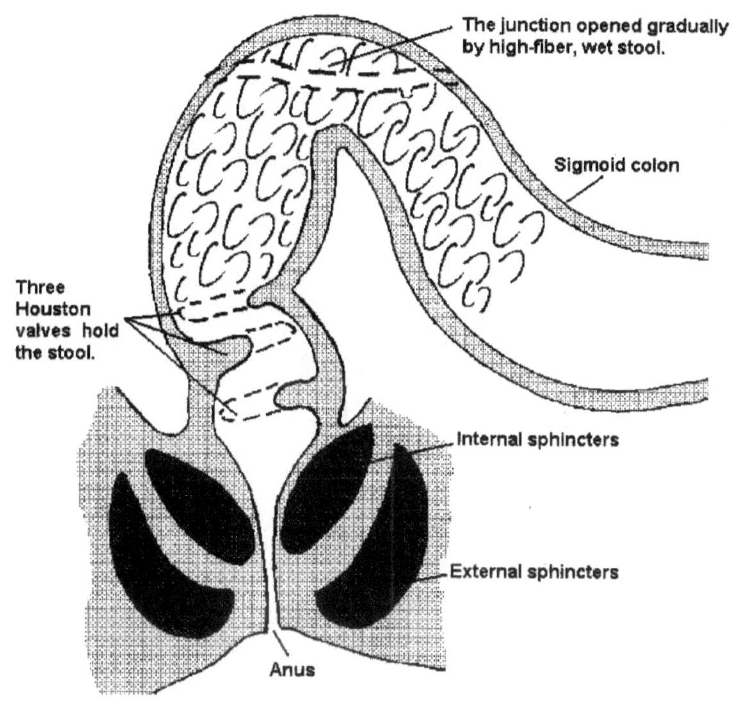

Figure 14: Rectosigmoid junction with a high-fiber, high-moisture stool.

Need a convincing experiment, a real teaching aid?

To demonstrate for yourself the advantages of fiber and moisture, do the following:

A. Obtain miller's bran from your natural health food store.

B. Remove the crust from two slices of bread. From one of the pieces, mold by hand a stool that resembles the one shown in figures 12 and 13. This simulates a high-protein-residue, low-moisture stool. While forming, think how much effort it's going to take to get this through the junction.

C. Place the other piece of bread on a plate in water 1/8 inch deep, sprinkle two tablespoons of miller's bran on top, and try to mold into a stool. It won't work. This stool (Figure 14) cannot be molded or compacted, so it will flow easily through any junction. That's it. It's this simple.

How doctors view the rectosigmoid junction and scoping the sigmoid colon

Like Mount Everest, one must attempt it because it's there.

When doctors examine the sigmoid colon with a sigmoidoscope (12" or longer rod with a viewing device attached to one end) they describe this curve, the rectosigmoid junction as **"tortuous to negotiate and only accomplished one half the time."** Their motto is "It is better to have scoped and failed than never to have scoped at all." When failing, they schedule a colonoscopy, which uses flexible tube. [End Notes 13]

Enlightenment

One can only surmise the advantages a doctor has with leverage, manipulation and strength to reach the sigmoid colon and go through to the descending colon with a sigmoidoscope. Yet, he only succeeds **50% of the time.** If we apply this information in the opposite direction to a stool that's hard, high in protein, and lacks flowability due to low fiber and moisture content, we soon realize what constipation really is.

Other problems the junction causes

Suppressing the urge to eliminate because of the pain, straining, time and effort due to this severe curve/junction will generally cause both short-term and long-term physical problems, such as:

- Increases time required to pass through the colon by backing up and drying out the entire system.

- Greatly increases elimination time and straining.

- Increases buildup of residue on the colon wall, contaminating the body's water supply.

- Increases the need for medication to cure constipation and the conditions it causes.

- Directly relates to any health condition found on pages 27-28.

16-How Fiber and Moisture Work

The rectum is normally empty. The exceptions are stools, extremely high in moisture and fiber that is soft enough to flow through the junction without the normal signals and are held in check by the Houston valves (Figure 14.)

Normally, cerebral signals are sent to the sigmoid colon and rectosigmoid junction to relax, straighten, and start contractions after a meal or on a full colon. (Notice a dog, that after eating, waits at the door because of this signal.)

If the correct consistency of fiber and moisture is present, the stool will flow through the junction into the rectum to await the desired signal. If however, fiber and moisture are lacking, nothing happens and your stool generally remains behind the sigmoid junction to await a bout of serious straining or a laxative to pass through the junction. **Constipation has arrived.**

Now arriving at the rectum

The rectum is engineered to accept the stool, store it until some convenient time later and above all not to leak. How does it do this? The healthy internal sphincter muscle (see Figure 15,) located in the rectum, automatically reacts and closes (continence.)

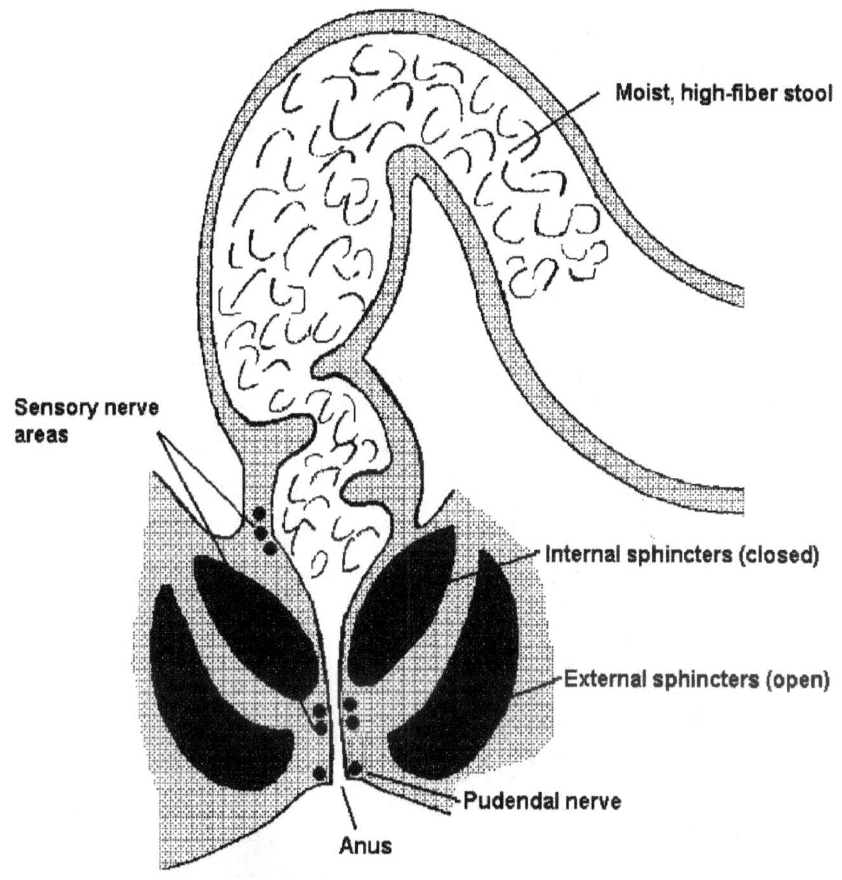

Figure 15: Internal sphincters reacting to a moist, high-fiber stool and closing (involuntary).

When a sufficient buildup of feces is detected in this area, which is rich in sensory nerve endings, the internal sphincter opens up and the contents of the rectum are released to the external sphincter muscle (Figure 16) for voluntary elimination. It's now time for you to decide whether to continue the conversation and squeeze the sphincter muscle harder or excuse yourself. [End Notes 14].

Below the external sphincter muscle in the anal canal is the pudendal nerve (Figure 16), which tells us the difference between gas and solids (most of the time.)

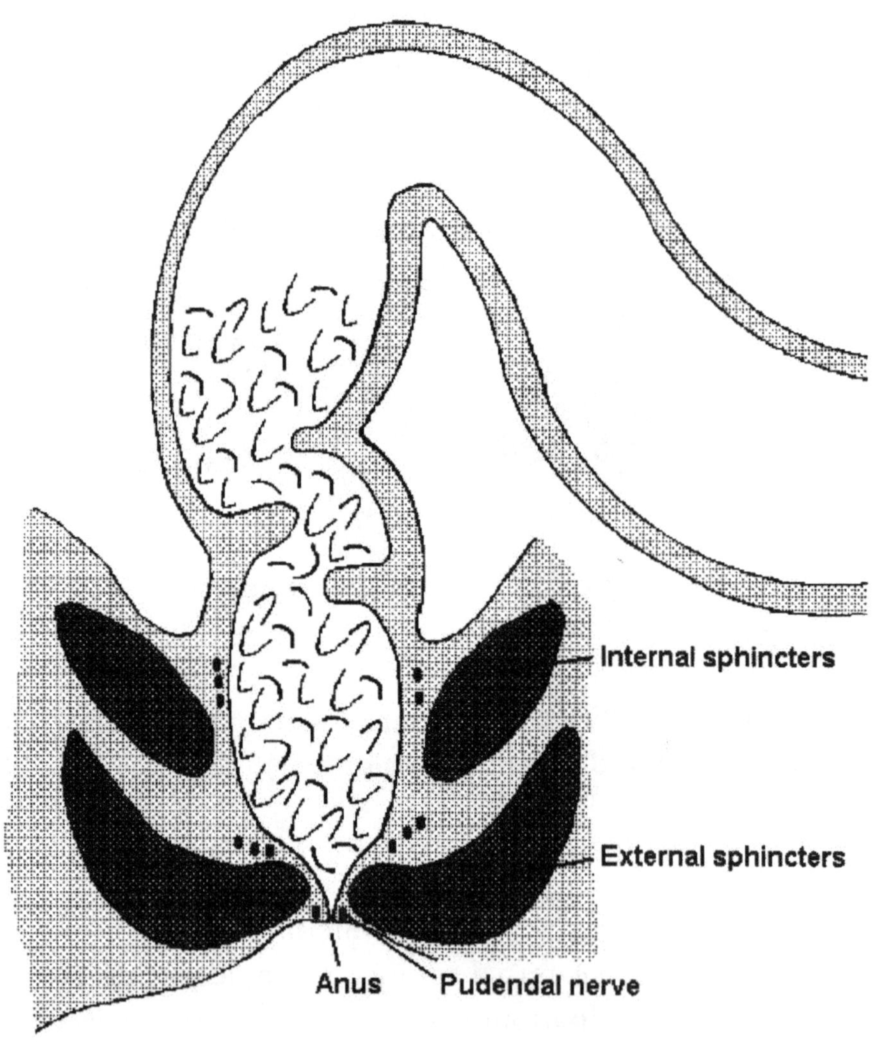

Figure 16: Internal sphincters reacting to the quantity of the stool and releasing to the external sphincters.

Finally, elimination

The anus at rest is a small slit. When eliminating it contracts, straightens and enlarges. The contractions are supplied by muscles in this rich sensory nerve area, awaiting that voluntary command.

The amount of feces eliminated may be as much as 2 feet in length, draining the entire descending colon if the correct amounts of soluble fiber, insoluble fiber and moisture are present.

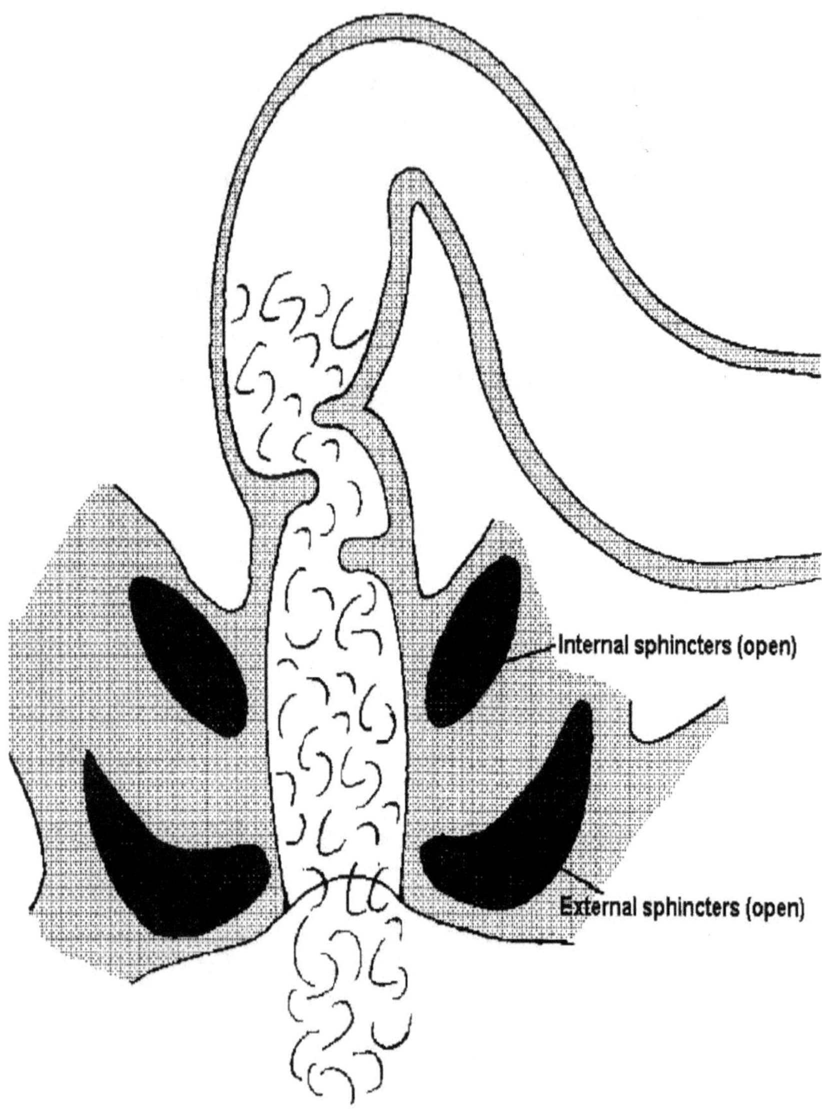

Figure 17: External sphincters opening in response to a voluntary command.

Digitation (The manual starter button)

This method can be used to induce muscle contractions manually and basically start all the actions the body starts automatically by gently massaging inside the anus, which contains all the sensitive nerve endings. This process can be useful to produce a stool on your timetable, reduce straining, or start what may not happen automatically. However, the correct fiber and moisture content must be present.

In Conclusion

All of the enclosed information was researched at the Scott Memorial Library at Thomas Jefferson University, a prestigious medical school in Philadelphia, Pennsylvania.

All the pertinent information reviewed reflected the same point of view regarding water and fiber. The author used the information and applied it in a practical way that would benefit everyone's understanding of a topic that's vitally important, but never discussed. The objective is to help you to lead a healthy life with abundant energy and without the fear of the numerous diseases that have been linked to poor colon health.

It's not much of a stretch for the imagination to view water and fiber as the main ingredients in a favorite recipe. Fail to measure one correctly and leave one ingredient almost out, then simmer, boil or bake too long, and the results can be

.....disastrous

In closing, I'd like to say that this message of water, fiber and transit time should be conveyed to everyone – parents to their kids and extended families, teachers to the students, coaches to athletes, and employers to employees for growth, survival, energy and a feeling of well-being and good health for all.

Appendixes

Points to remember

1. Plan the time to have a bowel movement. The best time is after a meal when natural signals are being sent to the colon for movement. Train the muscles involved to react at the same time every day, twice a day. Even if a stool is not produced, train the muscles to eliminate. In the beginning you will go back and forth between producing no stool, a constipated stool and a non-constipated stool. This is due to your colon's condition, food choices, and correct water and fiber intake. Soon a natural bodily habit will emerge.

2. Medication will have a direct bearing on producing a timely stool. Please see page 98, of the Appendix for some medications that can cause constipation. If you are not sure or have any questions, talk with your pharmacist.

3. Toilet accommodation's that do not allow total concentration are a leading factor in constipation. However, when correct water and fiber levels are reached, a bowel movement becomes almost as easy as urination.

4. Children should not have feet dangling from the toilet because it impairs adequate intra-abdominal pressure, which can be achieved only when feet contact the floor. Consider using a small bench or a stack of books under each foot. Make sure the knees are at least a foot apart from each other.

5. Postponing elimination results in drying the front of the stool in the rectosigmoid junction, which means you

will have to strain until the dried portion is passed, or you will have a bout of constipation.

6.   Stool color is helpful in determining if you have a healthy stool. Feces starts out as green in the cecum and ascending colon, then changes to light brown as it passes through the transverse colon and gradually loses moisture. Finally, it turns a darker brown as it loses more moisture in the descending colon.

7.   Gas in the colon will become almost odorless as fiber is increased and the colon loses its sidewall residue.

8.   Seeds that are eaten may swell, which is a natural part of their growth process. This happens in the colon due to the warm and moist conditions; they can create a blockage, leading to constipation.

9.   Conversation on this delicate topic may be best served by starting with the difference between soluble and insoluble fiber.

10. Your colon will occasionally take a day off; don't become that concerned.

11. It will be beneficial to have a general understanding of prebiotic and probiotic and how they affect your colon.

Foods and fiber – food for thought

The apple, the most versatile

Let's take a look at the common apple. The skin of an apple is a good source of insoluble fiber, supplying 2 to 3 grams. **However, the skin can cause constipation.** The inside provides soluble fiber, which is good for the fermentation cycle, encouraging moisture-grabbing bacteria to soften the stool and create carbon dioxide. This gas helps propels the stool forward. Another feature of the apple is its entrained water. A large apple will contain almost 6 ounces of entrained water. The apple is a great traveling companion, reducing the need for rest stops for urination.

Oatmeal, the super food

Oatmeal contains protein and ranks just behind fish in efficiency. It has 8 grams of insoluble fiber per half cup, plus 1 gram of soluble fiber, yet it contains only 200 calories and is low in fat. It is rich in vitamins E and B. Oatmeal will absorb and entrain water, and because of this ability will give you a full feeling to curb your appetite. Is it any wonder that healthy families were raised solely on three meals a day of oatmeal during the Great Depression?

Oatmeal is easy to use. Just put two handfuls in a bowl, cover with water and microwave for two minutes. Add fruit, bran, and skim milk if desired.

A hamburger and fries, America's favorite

A large hamburger has 580 calories and 34 grams of fat and 50 grams of protein. French fries contribute 530 more calories and 26 grams of fat. **Together, these provide less than 1 gram of soluble or insoluble fiber.**

Screening for colon problems

1. **Colonoscopy** gives the best view of the colon wall. It

uses a fiber-optic, lighted tube that is flexible. It is half an inch in diameter and 6 feet long. Using this tool, the doctor can examine the ascending, transverse, and descending colon for most conditions. If polyps are present, they can be removed for biopsy using the same tool. A colonoscopy cannot give an overall picture of the colon the way the virtual colonoscopy or barium enema can.

2.   The **virtual colonoscopy** provides a complete picture of the colon, is non-invasive, and requires no recovery time. It shows the shape, size and location of the colon and will identify the difficult areas and turns, especially the rectosigmoid junction. It gives an overview, so that you can adjust your water and fiber intake accordingly. However, if polyps are found, a colonoscopy must be scheduled to remove them.

3.   The **double-contrast barium enema** is the old style of a virtual colonoscopy, which is given in enema form. The enema is chemically treated so that colon abnormalities can be seen after being x-rayed. However, x-rays are difficult to read and require considerable expertise to evaluate. As with virtual colonoscopy, if any abnormalities are found, a colonoscopy is required for removal.

4.   A **proctosigmoidoscopy** uses a sigmoidoscope, which is a 12- to 24-inch fiber-optic, lighted tube that may be flexible or non-flexible. The sigmoidoscope is designed for finding polyps in the descending colon, sigmoid colon, rectosigmoid junction, rectum, and anal canal. These areas account for 80% of colon problems. The procedure is generally painless, although this depends on the

configuration at the junction. It is successful only half the time. Proctosigmoidoscopy can be performed in the doctor's office, and if polyps are found they can be removed.

Products and books used by the author

The items mentioned here are not endorsed, nor does the author receive compensation from any company.

Foods

Miller's bran (not a brand name) is the result of milling of wheat. It's usually found in a barrel in the health food store. It is relatively inexpensive. A pound will last for a week or two.

Oatmeal (unprocessed) is also found at the health food store (also can be found in certain supermarkets.) It is about the same price as miller's bran, and a pound will also last for a week or two.

All Bran and All Bran Extra are two Kellogg's cereals that provide 9 to 13 grams of insoluble fiber per serving. You'll find them in the supermarket in the cereal aisle, on the top or bottom shelf, out of sight.

Fiber One from General Mills contains 14 grams of insoluble fiber per serving. It's also in your supermarket cereal section, on the top shelf.

Shredded Wheat and Bran from Post contains 7 grams of insoluble fiber per serving. Look for it in the supermarket cereal aisle on the top and middle shelves.

Kashi, from Kashi Company, is actually four or five different types of cereals, some containing 8 to 10 grams or more of insoluble fiber. Kashi combines many types of insoluble fiber. It can be found in the health food section or cereal aisle of your supermarket or health food store.

Weetabix (a brand name) is found in health food stores. It contains a sufficient amount of insoluble fiber to be helpful.

Prunes are a good source of soluble fiber and a natural laxative that works extremely well. A daily requirement need be only 2 or 3.

Apples are another good source of soluble fiber that works well. Try different kinds, but **watch out** after high-protein meals. Apples may lead to a good fermentation rate (gas,) which may cause abdominal cramps if it gets caught behind high-protein, 3-foot stools that can seal and trap the gas.

Lentil soup or any bean soup is a good source of insoluble (7 grams) and soluble fiber. There are many recipes. Cabbage soup is another good source of soluble fiber.

Psyllium seed husks (commercial insoluble fiber that absorbs vast amounts of moisture, see pages 46) is found in health food stores as Yerba Prima, in many colon care products, and in your drug store as Metamucil. The laxative section of the store will have other products containing psyllium seed husks. However, a good psyllium seed product will not cause discomfort, as long as you implement it into your diet **slowly** and with the correct amount of water.

Books

In addition to the books listed in the End Notes section of this book, Stephen Fisher's Colon Cancer & The Polyps Connection (1995, Fisher Books, Tucson, Arizona) gives another informative view on this topic.

Laxatives and Enemas

Any laxative containing psyllium seed husks is recommended. These laxatives bulk the stool to take advantage of the body's normal functions (the colon pump.) The Food and Drug Administration is banning certain laxatives because they increase the risk of colon cancer. Consult your pharmacist about laxative ingredients. Fleet or other small disposable enemas are useful after long trips to add moisture to the rectosigmoid junction to produce a stool.

Conversion chart: ounces to grams

OZ.		gm.
0		0
1		
2		50
3		
4		100
5		150
6		
7		200
8		
9		250
10		
11		300
12		350
13		
14		400
15		
16		450

Medications associated with constipation

Many commonly used medications can cause constipation. These include amantidine, amitriptyline opiates, diuretics, iron supplements, Diltiazem, Nifedipine, Verpamil, non-steroidal anti-inflammatory agents, Biperiden, benztropine, benzhexol, Desipramine, and Doxepin.

***It's important to know the facts about what you're taking. Beware of the vicious cycle – prescription or over-the-counter constipating drugs followed by laxatives, which is destructive to your body rhythm. Once your system is out of sync, and without knowledge of what's going on, you suffer from drug dependence and ill health for life. If you are not sure about a medication, check with your pharmacist. ***

Diseases associated with less than 25 to 35 grams of insoluble fiber

This section describes some of the many diseases associated with inadequate insoluble fiber in the diet. Not included, however, are the illnesses that may be compounded by different combinations of medications and vitamins.

Anemia

Millions of Americans suffer from anemia, a reduction in either the number of red blood cells or the amount of hemoglobin in the blood. This results in a decrease in the amount of oxygen that the blood is able to carry. As a result, less energy is available to perform our daily tasks, both physically and mentally. [End Notes 15]

The symptoms: weakness, fatigue, coldness of the extremities, depression, dizziness, brittle nails, soreness in the mouth and, in women, cessation of menstruation.

Breast cancer

Generally caused by a diet high in fat and low in fiber that allows the body to produce more estrogen, which results in unrestricted cellular growth. It's also worth considering that the lack of fiber to absorb contaminants means they are absorbed by the soft tissues of the breasts, which may account for breast cancer showing up in over weight males.

Chronic diarrhea

A condition resulting from the body's attempt to rid itself of irritation caused by persistent intestinal parasites or bacterial infection, which thrive in the residue left on the colon wall when a low-fiber diet is consumed.

Crohn's disease

Inflammation of the alimentary tract, mouth to anus. A general breakdown of the entire system. Best described as open sores, causing stomach pain, fever, and diarrhea.

Colorectal cancer

A cancer that is found in the large colon and rectum. Common symptoms are rectal bleeding, blood in the stool, and changes in bowel habits (persistent diarrhea and/or constipation.)

Colon polyps

Tumors on the side walls of the colon that may grow to the size of a baseball and are caused by rotting, stagnating feces. They are only discovered during a routine colon examination (colonoscopy or virtual colonoscopy), but may cause rectal bleeding, cramping, or abdominal pain. It is believed that colorectal cancer begins from polyps. A greater percentage of polyps are found in the descending colon.

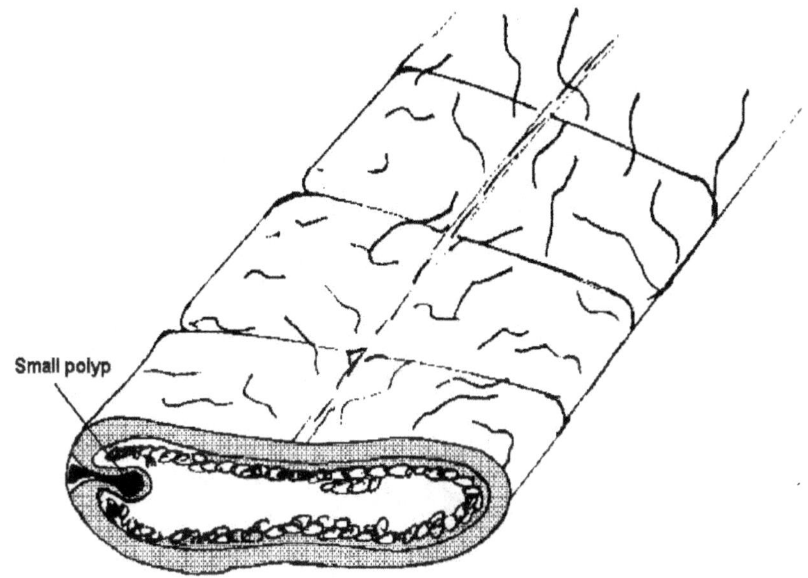

Figure 18: Flat, unhealthy colon with small polyp.

Coronary heart disease

The arteries that supply blood to the heart have narrowed by fat being stored on their walls, called cholesterol. As a result, the amount of blood they supply to the heart is insufficient to provide the oxygen the heart needs. This is a direct result of a low fiber, high protein, fatty diet.

Diverticula

It is the herniation of the mucosa (colon lining) because of defects in the diseased or rotting lining. Without sufficient fiber to soften and bulk, stools are harder to pass. Now, increased pressure is required to force small portions of hard, dry stool through the bowel. This rise in pressure can cause pouches to form at weak points in the colon wall. [End Notes 16]

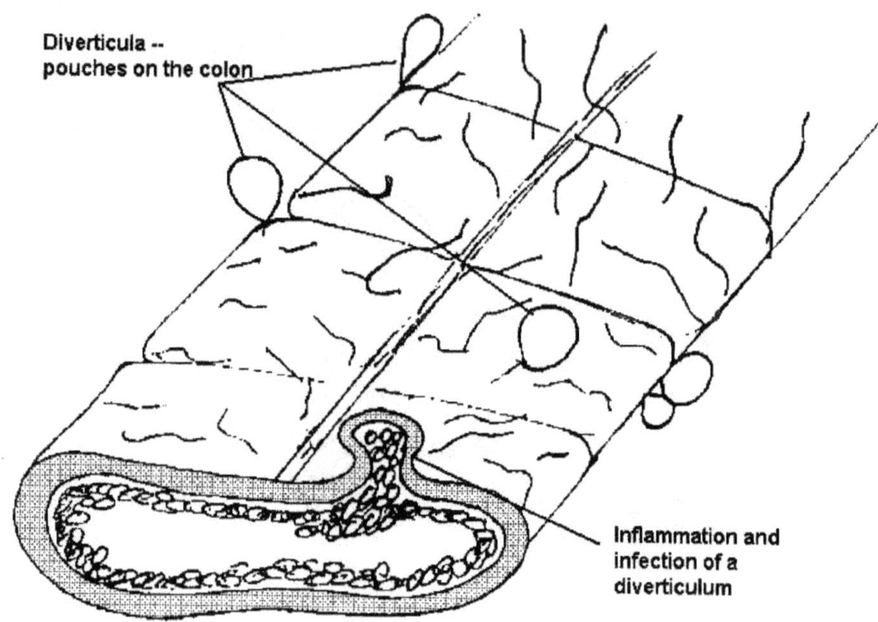

Figure 19: Diverticulosis is many pouches in the colon wall.

Diverticulosis

Term for having the diverticula on the colon. The barium enema and virtual colonoscopy are useful for detecting this condition.

Diverticulitis

It is the inflammation and infection of the pouch (diverticula) by rotting feces on the inside. The most common symptom is a crampy pain usually in the left side of the abdomen, associated with nausea and fever. It also can be a cause of chronic diarrhea as the body tries to expel the irritation.

Gallstones

A stone formed in the gallbladder or a bile duct, caused by an excess of what should have been absorbed by fiber. Instead, it's stored by the body as stones, becoming another storage problem and may cause severe stomach pain.

Gout

A common type of arthritis that attacks joints in the form of swelling, stiffness and decreased range of motion. It happens when a buildup of purines crystallize and store themselves in joints.

Hiatal hernia

The stomach herniates, goes through the lining into the thorax, allowing stomach acid to come back up the throat causing a condition called heartburn. The symptoms are belching, a burning sensation, and discomfort behind the breastbone.

Hypothyroidism

An underproduction of thyroid hormone. Symptoms of this include fatigue, loss of appetite, inability to tolerate cold, weight gain, painful premenstrual periods, a milky discharge from the breasts, fertility problems, muscle weakness, muscle cramps, dry and scaly skin, yellow-orange coloration in the skin, hair loss, recurrent infections, constipation, depression, and difficulty concentrating. The most common symptoms are fatigue and intolerance to cold. [End Notes 17]

Irritable bowel syndrome

The immediate conditions caused by low fiber and moisture in the colon. The common conditions include constipation, diarrhea, nausea, flatulence and bloating, all of which are related to stagnating, rotting material on the colon wall. This condition may also be called a spastic colon. It's the most common digestive disorder and, in fact, four out of every 5 adults have symptoms.

Myasthenia gravis

A weakness of muscle.

Multiple sclerosis (MS)

A progressive degenerative disorder of the central nervous system, including the brain, the optic nerve and spinal cord. The disease affects various parts of the nervous system by destroying the myelin sheaths that cover the nerves and leaving scar tissue called plaques, ultimately resulting in destruction of the nerves. This process is known as sclerosis.

The symptoms are mood swings, depression, and eye problems, such as blurred or double vision. Other symptoms include a feeling of tingling and/or numbness, especially in the hands and feet, loss of balance and/or coordination, muscular stiffness, nausea and vomiting, slurred speech, tremors, a vague feeling of weakness and/or fatigue, difficulty in breathing and, for men, impotence. [End Notes 18]

Paget's disease

Destruction of bone by the body, followed by the replacement with overdeveloped light, soft, porous bone, associated with deformities. The symptoms are pain in the affected bones that becomes more extreme over time, unexplained bone fractures, hearing loss, headaches, ringing in the ears.

Pernicious anemia

The defective production of red blood cells, which directly affects the absorption of vitamin B. Vitamin B maintains the health of nerves, skins, eyes, hair and liver. Vitamin B is also involved in energy production. **Alzheimer's disease can be a result of a deficiency of vitamin B**.

Pulmonary embolism

The plugging of pulmonary arteries with fragments of a thrombus most frequently from the leg, after an operation.

Rheumatoid Arthritis

Swelling and stiffness of joints found at the knees, wrists, elbows fingers, toes, hip, and shoulders.

Ulcerative Colitis

The colon lining (mucosa) develops ulcers. This may cause diarrhea, bloating and blood in the stool.

The enema

The enema is of no use, because water cannot remove oils and sticky protein. To see for yourself, try running water over a plate with eggs residue on the surface or a bowl coated with salad oil.

Colonoscopy prep: cleaning out the colon

Follow your Doctor's instructions.

About the author

Emmanuel Enderlein grew up in manufacturing America. At the age of sixteen, he started as an iron worker in a Philadelphia Foundry, where he spent summers and holiday vacations working as a laborer. He graduated from Waynesburg College and enlisted in the Pennsylvania Air National Guard. Upon returning to civilian employment he entered a foundry apprentice program, which entailed working at every level of the operation – pouring metal, furnace operations, plant maintenance, and the supporting technical courses.

He attended night school at the University of Pennsylvania, Wharton School to further his education in management. These activities contributed to the H. G. Enderlein Company being recognized as the casting vendor of the year in 1976 by Carrier Air Conditioning.

In 1988, Mr. Enderlein was awarded U.S. Patent 4,767,278 in Marine Propulsion, which was a result of his combined knowledge in metallurgy and engineering that produced a low-cost, high-strength propeller for small boats.

His current interests center around health, running, and landscape design.

The author's daily fiber intake

This is not a diet, although care and consideration should be taken on the amount and quality of other foods after correct fiber intake is achieved. The amount of soluble and insoluble fiber needed will vary from person to person.

For breakfast, I never consider any protein products with the exception of skim milk. I have a cup and a half of cereal with milk, which provides 9 grams per cup or approximently 14 grams of insoluble fiber. I purchase cereal with many types of grains. You may want to check that out under ingredients. Each fiber grain does something different, I also find that it works more effectively to sprinkle approximately another 4 grams of miller's bran (2 teaspoons), with fruit. During the morning, I have an apple or a couple of prunes. I do enjoy a doughnut with a cup of coffee every once in a while.

For lunch, I like soup, such as cabbage, lentil or bean, or a fruit if I'm in a hurry. Before dinner, it's psyllium seed husks (a full teaspoon or two) with two glasses of water. The psyllium seed creates a full feeling, thus reducing my appetite.

Dinner, with my personal daily fiber requirements met, is the standard American menu. My favorite is a taco salad, the one topped with chili, which is a great help and has fiber, the occasional hamburger and fries, spaghetti and meatballs, pork and sauerkraut, and especially fish.

End notes

1.   (p. 15) H. Trowell, Dietary Fibre, fibre-depleted foods and disease. 1985. Academic Press Harcourt, Brace, Jovanovich. London, Orlando, San Diego, New York. page 14.

2.   (p. 15) R. Ballentine, Radical Healing. Harmony Books, 1999. New York. page 280.

3.   (p. 16) same as note 2.

4.   (p. 19) R. Gray, The Colon Health Book. 1991. Emerald, Reno. page 16.

5.   (p. 20) H. Trowell, Dietary Fibre, fibre-depleted foods and disease. 1985. Academic Press Harcourt, Brace, Jovanovich. London, Orlando, San Diego, New York. page 6.

6.   (p. 21) H. Trowell, Dietary Fibre, fibre-depleted foods and disease. 1985. Academic Press Harcourt, Brace, Jovanovich. London, Orlando, San Diego, New York. page 7.

7.   (p. 24) R. Ballentine, Radical Healing. Harmony Books, 1999. New York. page 296.

8.   (p. 27) Cummings et al. 1978a. Cited by A. Stephen, in H. Trowell and D. Burkitt, eds., Dietary Fibre, fibre-depleted foods and disease. 1985. Academic Press Harcourt, Brace, Jovanovich. London, Orlando, San Diego, New York. page 137.

9. (p. 27) Collier's Encyclopedia. 1989. Macmillan Educational Col., New York. page 398.

10. (p. 28) Dimock, 1937. Cited by A. Stephen, in H. Trowell and D. Burkitt, eds., Dietary Fibre, fibre-depleted foods and disease. 1985. Academic Press Harcourt, Brace, Jovanovich. London, Orlando, San Diego, New York. page 137.

11. (p. 49) H. Janowitz, Your gut feeling. 1999. University Park Press, New York. page 111.

12. (p. 57) W. Thompson, The irritable gut. 1979. University Park Press, New York. page 18.

13. (p. 63) W. Thompson, The irritable gut. 1979. University Park Press, New York. page 58.

14. (p. 66) W. Thompson, The irritable gut. 1979. University Park Press, New York. page 17.

15. (p. 77) J. Balch and P. Balch, Prescription for nutritional healing. 1997. Avery Publishing, New York. page 174.

16. (p. 79) J. Balch and P. Balch, Prescription for nutritional healing. 1997. Avery Publishing, New York. page 328.

17. (p. 80) J. Balch and P Balch, Prescription for nutritional healing. 1997. Avery Publishing, New York. page 334.

18. (p. 81) J. Balch and P Balch, Prescription for nutritional healing. 1997. Avery Publishing, New York.

page 392.